Bea Northcott
Janette Helm

Untapped Options

**Building Links Between
Marketing and Human Resources
to Achieve Organizational Goals
in Health Care**

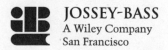
JOSSEY-BASS
A Wiley Company
San Francisco

Health Forum, Inc.
An American Hospital Association Company
CHICAGO
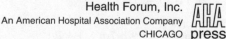

Manufactured in the United States of America on Lyons Falls
Turin Book. This paper is acid-free and 100 percent totally
chlorine-free.

Library of Congress Cataloging-in-Publication Data

Northcott, Bea.
        Untapped options : building links between marketing and
    human resources to achieve organizational goals in healthcare /
    Bea Northcott, Janette Helm.
            p.   cm.
        Includes bibliographical references and index.
        ISBN 0-7879-5537-X (hardcover)
        1. Health facilities—Personnel management. 2. Medical care—
    Marketing. I. Helm, Janette. II. Title.
    RA971.35.N67 2000
    362.1'068'3—dc21   00-022052

FIRST EDITION
HB Printing   10 9 8 7 6 5 4 3 2 1

Contents

List of Figures and Table   xi

About the Authors   xiii

Acknowledgments   xv

1. The Untapped Option   1
    New Pressures in the Workplace
    Positive Work Environments
    • For-Profit and Not-for-Profit Organizations
    • Financial Performance and Employee Satisfaction
    • Characteristics of Positive Work Environments
    • Obstacles to Creating Positive Work Environments
    Conclusion: Moving Beyond the Common
    Case Study: An Employer of Choice, Eli Lilly and Company

2. Creating and Evaluating Mission, Vision, and Values   23
    Distinctions Between Mission, Vision, and Values
    • Mission
    • Vision
    • Values
    Conclusion
    Case Study: A Vision-Driven Move at Methodist Hospital of
      Indiana, Inc.

3. Implementing Mission, Vision, and Values   47
    Developing Strategy from Mission, Vision, and Values
    From Philosophy to Fulfillment
    The Leadership Void

Doing Well for Yourself by Doing Good for the Organization
Case Study: Living the Mission at McMurry Publishing, Inc.
- Mission and Values
- Monday Morning Meetings
- Independent Decision Making
- Evaluation System
- Open-Book Management and Profit Sharing

4. Linking Human Resources and Marketing   71
Out with the Old
The Current View
In with the New
Intellectual Capital
Human Resources and Marketing: Similarities
- Customer Service Excellence
- Alignment
- Customer Focus
- Internal Communication
- Working with Other Departments
- Similar Tools
Human Resources and Marketing: Differences
Negative Similarities
Benefits of Working Together
- A Profitable Venture
- An Exchange of Information
- Cross-Selling the Organization
- Developing Core Competencies
- Satisfied Employees, Satisfied Customers
Accreditation Issues
Models for Working Together
Case Study: One Model for Integration at 1st Community Bank
    and Trust

5. Recruiting and Motivating a Changing Workforce   97
The Changing Workplace
- Worker Expectations

- Recruiting Students
- Recruiting Experienced Workers
- Recruiting the Right People

Measuring Behavior
- Performance Appraisals
- Behavioral Objectives
- Rewards and Recognition

Diversity Issues
- Generation X
- Baby Boomers
- Traditionalists

Work and Personal Issues

Keeping Employees Motivated in Difficult Times

Implications of Health Promotion for the Workplace

Case Study: Following the Disney Model at University of
    Chicago Hospitals
- Hiring Practices
- Learning Academy—Continuing Education
- Summary

6. Hiring the Right People   121
    Demographic Shifts in the Workplace
    Characteristics of Fulfilling Work
    Characteristics of the Right Employees for Your Organization
    Recruitment
    - Written and Internet Advertisements
    - Job Fairs
    - Hiring from Within the Organization
    - Executive Search Firms

    The Interview
    - Behavioral Interview Questions
    - Identifying Potential Problem Behavior
    - Questions the Best Candidates Ask
    - Interview Teams
    - Scoring Grids
    - Follow-up

Promotion of Organizational Values
Case Studies
- Rosenbluth Travel
- McMurry Publishing

7. Training and Performance Development   139

Levels of Training and Development
Justifying Training Programs
Defining the Need
Internal Versus External Trainers
Defining Behavioral Expectations of Employees
- The Initial Interview
- The Orientation Program
- Preceptor or Mentor Programs
- Performance Appraisals
Empowering Employees
Defining Terminology
Performance Development
Expanding the Boundaries of Training
Measuring Employee Satisfaction
Case Study: People-Centered Teams Healing the Workplace
   at St. Charles Medical Center

8. Structuring Employee Benefits   159

Creating and Maintaining the Salary and Benefits Package
- Health Benefits
- Sick Days and Well Days
- Health Promotion
- Flexible Benefits
- Flextime
- Dependent Care
- Opportunities for Advancement
- Compensation—Not Just Money
Balancing Work and Personal Life
Aligning Human Resources and Marketing

People Make the Place

Case Study: A Culture Restructured at WakeMed

- Components of the Program
- Recognition
- Other Changes
- Ongoing Commitment

9. Marketing   179

How Consumers Choose a Provider

Perception Versus Reality

Internal Communications

- Employee Communications
- Communication with Other Internal Audiences
- New Ideas

External Communications

- How to Communicate
- The Costs and Benefits of Advertising

Positive Promotion

Marketing as an Operational Support

Other Marketing Functions

Customer Satisfaction

One-to-One Marketing

The Long-Term Impact of Marketing Communications

Case Study: The 90-Day Checkup of Baptist Hospital
of Pensacola

10. Beginning the Change Process   205

Leading People Through the Process of Change

Report from the Future

Learn from the Best

Looking Within Ourselves to Create Change

Index   213

List of Figures and Table

Figure 1.1   Model of the Untapped Option: Human   3
Resources and Marketing Linked

Figure 2.1   Mission Statement Guidelines   27

Figure 2.2   Steps in the Vision Creation Process   34

Figure 3.1   Questions for the Strategy Development   50
Session

Figure 3.2   Seven C's of the Strategic Commitment   52
Process

Figure 3.3   Additional Necessities to Gain Employee   53
Commitment

Figure 3.4   Behavioral Trust and Change Program   59

Figure 5.1   Johnson Memorial Hospital Award Programs   107

Table 7.1   Traditional Versus Performance Approach   152
to Training and Development

Figure 8.1   Two Successful Health Promotion Programs   164

Figure 8.2   Innovative Health Promotion: 165
Massage Therapy

About the Authors

Bea Northcott is president of Triple Impact, a marketing, training, and human resources consulting company. She has worked for both proprietary and not-for-profit hospitals in marketing, public relations, and business development. She is a Certified Health Care Manager and 1997 graduate of Leadership Johnson County. She is a member of the Society for Healthcare Strategy and Market Development and an officer of the Indiana Society for Healthcare Planning and Marketing. She achieved the Certified Level of the American Society for Health Care Marketing and Public Relations' Professional Achievement Program in 1993. She has a bachelor's degree in journalism and French from Butler University, Indianapolis, and a master's degree in human resources management from Kennedy-Western University.

Janette Helm is an organizational development consultant for St. Vincent Hospital and Health Services in Indianapolis. She has fourteen years' experience in health care education and development. She is a Registered Nurse (RN), a Certified Health Education Specialist (CHES), and a Certified Health Care Manager. She is a member of the American Society for Healthcare Human Resources Administration, the Indiana Society for Healthcare Education and Training, and the Society for Public Health Education and past president of the Indiana Association of Health Educators. She has a bachelor's and a master's degree in community health education from Ball State University, Muncie, Indiana, and a nursing degree from Anderson University, Anderson, Indiana. She has presented educational sessions at state and national conferences on such topics as health promotion, developing community partnerships, and building employee morale.

Acknowledgments

We would like to thank the individuals who were willing to share the experiences of their organizations. These case studies help us all understand the inherent obstacles and the achievements that are possible when we make the effort to link human resources and marketing: Don Goeb, Martyn Howgill, Bill Loveday, Candice Lang, Preston McMurry, Christopher McMurry, Stephanie Powell, Quint Studer, Jill Bloom, Rebecca Christian, JoAnn Shaw, and Bill Carmichael.

We are deeply grateful to those who reviewed the manuscript, provided feedback, offered ideas or a sounding board, or assisted us in other ways: Reginald M. Ballantyne III, Steve Ellson, Tom Owens, Sheila Ridner, Robert Riney, Anne Streeter, Sue Kuryla, Carrie Meyer, Chris Meyer, and Michael P. Scott.

Rick Hill and Ron Mills provided editorial assistance, guidance, and support, and we thank them.

And finally, and most important, thank you to our husbands, Ron Branson and Chris Northcott, who endured the time it took away from other responsibilities and supported us throughout this process.

Chapter One

The Untapped Option

Hospitals and other health care organizations have been talking about cost containment since the late 1970s. Yet health care costs continue to rise faster than inflation, businesses are constantly looking for ways to reduce their health care expenditures, managed care and other insurance companies continue to search for ways to reduce their costs, and consumers still want the highest-quality care exactly when they need it at a low price.

It seems that we have exhausted all options to control costs. We enter into contracts with group purchasing organizations to take advantage of volume discounts. We ask our department heads to reduce expenses whenever possible, even tying this goal to incentive payments. We reduce our wage and benefits budgets through attrition, layoffs, restructuring, or contract employment opportunities. We ask our employees to do more with less and do more complex tasks in less time.

Yet costs continue to escalate. We find it more and more difficult to attract, train, and retain employees qualified to perform both clinical and customer service duties. And we spend more and more money to attract new customers through promotional efforts.

Hospitals began years ago as charitable entities performing good works for the benefit of society. Today, it is an industry that accounts for more than 15 percent of the gross national product.

According to Brian D. Wong, partner and worldwide director of health care strategy for Arthur Andersen, "As a $1.3 trillion industry, healthcare is the fourth-largest economy in the world. But consumers and industry leaders alike see it as an industry that is constrained—without enough resources to go around. The root of the problem, however, isn't in a shortage of resources, but rather a misallocation of the resources that are available. This has occurred because leaders do not understand their core business" (Mycek, 1998, p. 27).

It seems that one option we haven't fully explored is right under our noses, perhaps too obvious to see. That option is to work within our own organizations to integrate certain functions that can maximize our most important resources—our employees and patients. The best part about this untapped option is that it is not a new management fad to implement; it is a natural extension of our organization's mission, vision, and values—our core business. Properly implemented, it can result in not only improved performance, but also increased patient satisfaction, increased employee satisfaction, and greater financial security for our organizations.

The untapped option is to link human resources (HR) and marketing functions to achieve organizational goals. This means not only having the employees in these two traditionally separate departments begin working more closely together, but also to have those employees work together with operational departments to improve operational performance.

Many people, the authors included, believe that the acts of employees are fully representative of the company's treatment of them. The untapped option is based on the assumption that satisfied employees are more productive and will provide better service to patients. It means treating our employees the way we want them to treat our patients. It means treating people right.

The model for the untapped option is this: Employees (including volunteers and physicians) are in large part responsible for an organization's reputation. Employees provide the care to patients and family members. The clinical outcome coupled with the performance of that treatment creates the image that a patient has of both the institution and its employees. Figure 1.1 shows a graphic model of the untapped option.

Figure 1.1 Model of the Untapped Option: Human Resources and Marketing Linked.

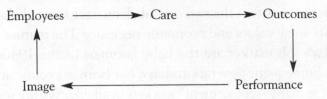

Employees who are supported in their work and clearly know the organization's goals and their role in achieving those goals can create the image and reputation that the organization wishes to achieve.

New Pressures in the Workplace

Most business owners, stockholders, hospital administrators, board members, and managers would agree that the two most valuable assets of any business are its employees and customers. Hiring, training, and retaining the employees who will make your business successful and treating your customers well so they will return are vitally important responsibilities for the manager, regardless of the industry or the size of the organization.

There are a variety of old and new pressures on health care organizations today that make employee relations a significant factor in an organization's ability to meet both financial and nonfinancial (customer satisfaction) goals. Some of these pressures come from the new generation of American workers, who not only are fewer in number, but also have different career and personal goals than previous generations. Other pressures come from new technology and our transformation from a manufacturing economy to a service economy and information society.

Because of these pressures it is necessary for health care organizations to reevaluate their ideas on employee satisfaction, productivity, and organizational performance. In their book *Re-inventing the Corporation*, Naisbitt and Aburdene (1985) say we are living in a rare time in history when the two crucial elements for social change are present—new values and economic necessity. The mature workers in today's job market are the baby boomers of the 1940s to the 1960s. Subsequent generations have not been as prolific and there are not as many "replacement" workers available. We are seeing the lowest unemployment rates ever in some portions of the country and low unemployment nationwide. With fewer potential employees in the job market, attracting the most qualified candidate for a particular job and retaining the valuable employees we already have become more important.

"Most corporations have gotten used to the comfort of operating in a buyer's market in labor, having their pick of many competent, qualified applicants for each job. Corporations will aggressively compete for fewer first-rate employees. The most talented people will be attracted to those corporations that succeed in re-inventing themselves into companies that are great places to work for because the people in them grow personally while contributing to the company" (p. 16).

Not only are there fewer employees waiting in the wings, but younger employees have a different attitude toward work than their parents and grandparents. "Generation X" employees are less willing to make personal sacrifices for their employers and are less likely to remain with the same employer for decades as their grandparents did. Employees are increasingly looking for ways to balance their work and personal lives. "GenXers" are people who intuitively "know that work should be fun and that it should be related to the other parts of their lives" (p. 5).

Finally, in a service economy and an information society, human resources become more important. In service industries such as health care, employees are directly responsible for the provision of the service and the customer's satisfaction. In a service industry, the person providing the service and the service itself are indistinguishable. Health care organizations depend on their employees' ability to process information and make split-second decisions. You must nurture employees to develop new and different skills to help the organization succeed and ensure that they will stay with the organization so that you can reap the benefits of that knowledge. The competition among employers to hire the best and brightest will only become more intense.

Training dissatisfied employees only to have them take their knowledge to another organization is both frustrating and costly. Not only have you lost your training investment, but you must also hire and train a new employee to replace the old one. Telecommunications company MCI learned in an employee study that in the first three months, a new hire accomplishes only 60 percent as much as an experienced worker and serves customers less well (Shellenbarger, 1998, p. B1).

Naisbitt and Aburdene (1985, p. 4) wrote, "In the new information society, human capital has replaced dollar capital as the strategic resource. People and profits are inexorably linked."

Positive Work Environments

Identifying and creating positive work environments that will attract and satisfy the best employees is more difficult to put into practice than to discuss. But it is critical to future survival. Naisbitt and Aburdene contend, "In an information society, human resources are any organization's competitive edge. American business has given this concept a kind of obligatory lip service in the past. Now it is time to understand the practical side: We will not see profits grow if we do not learn how to grow people" (p. 11).

For-Profit and Not-for-Profit Organizations

The management of a publicly traded company reports to its stockholders. The management of a not-for-profit organization reports to its stakeholders, such as its membership, donors, and the community at large. While the for-profit corporation is responsible for maximizing stockholders' investments, the not-for-profit organization is responsible to its constituents to responsibly allocate limited resources to serve its community. Like publicly traded companies, not-for-profit organizations such as hospitals need to make a profit to remain in business.

Historically, health care organizations have had the trust and confidence of their community residents who expect that the organization will act with integrity and in the community's best interest. However, this has changed in the past few years as health care organizations have begun acting more and more like corporations. The general public often believes that not-for-profit hospitals are, in fact, for-profit because of their behavior. The inaccurate perception of a health care organization's tax status is important not because for-profit hospitals are inherently bad and not-for-profit hospitals are inherently good. It is important because it emphasizes the point that not-for-profit hospitals have forgotten their core business.

A company's primary business is not to make or keep its employees happy. However, there is a significant correlation between happy employees and corporate financial performance. Many studies have been done with publicly traded companies to assess the correlation between employee job satisfaction and financial performance. Few have been done with not-for-profit organizations. Businesses that want to succeed in the future, whether for-profit or not-for-profit, need to understand and embrace this concept.

Financial Performance and Employee Satisfaction

There have been many studies that show a direct correlation between corporate profits and positive employee work environments.

A study of 968 large- and medium-sized firms in 35 U.S. industries looked at accounting profits, productivity, employee turnover, and human resource practices. "A solid relationship was found between the best HR practices and reduced turnover and increased employee productivity. Further, those practices enhanced profitability and market value of the firms studied. A high-quality, highly motivated workforce is hard for competition to replicate. It is an advantage that improves organizational performance, and it comes from effective HR management" (Mathis and Jackson, 1997, p. 592, quoting M. Zigarelli in "Human Resources and the Bottom Line," *Academy of Management Executive*, May 1996).

A 1984 study conducted by Patrick McVeigh, a stockbroker for Franklin Research and Development, compared the 70 publicly traded companies on the "100 Best Companies to Work for in America" list with Standard and Poor's 500. McVeigh used growth in profits over time and increase in stock price as his measurement tools. The study was reported in *A Great Place to Work* by Levering (1988, p. 259), who said, "The results were spectacular. Over the previous decade, the 100 Best companies outperformed the S&P 500 by a wide margin. The 100 Best companies were more than twice as profitable as the average of the S&P 500."

It was not that more profitable companies could afford to treat their employees better, he said, but that in each organization, positive employee relations and a positive work environment were, and always had been, a conscious decision.

Levering went on to quote several other, similar studies, all of which showed a significant correlation between increased financial performance and positive work environments. However, he said, "The research does not prove that good employers always perform better. Nor does it indicate that companies that exploit their workers never profit. But the research demonstrates that in general, the better employers enjoy more financial success than their competitors. I could find no study that could be used to argue the opposite viewpoint—that bad or mediocre employers perform better financially than good employers" (p. 262).

Standard indicators of job satisfaction among the many studies quoted in Levering's book include turnover rates, absenteeism rates, accident rates, and number of grievances filed by employees.

Research by Victor Vroom in the early 1960s showed that most people assume there is a connection between job satisfaction and job performance. The evidence Vroom collected in his research led him to conclude that there is a "consistent negative relationship between job satisfaction and the probability of resignation. This relationship appears when scores on job satisfaction are obtained from individuals and used to predict subsequent voluntary dropouts and when mean scores on job satisfaction of organizational units are correlated with turnover rates for these units" (Levering, 1988, p. 168).

He found a less consistent negative relationship between job satisfaction and absences. However, the relationship was most consistent when the frequency of unexcused absences was measured rather than actual lost work days.

Turnover, absenteeism, accidents, and grievances each have significant financial implications for a company. When factoring in the cost of recruiting and training a new worker, hiring a replacement worker, lost productivity, and other indirect costs, one can see that the cost of turnover is high. Avoidance of these costs will result in better financial performance. Many hospitals do not track turnover or absenteeism rates so they don't know exactly how much these indicators of employee dissatisfaction are costing.

Job satisfaction has also been shown to have an effect on customer satisfaction. More satisfied customers can result in more business for an organization, thus enhancing profitability. Also, more satisfied customers will share their experiences with other potential customers, enhancing an organization's marketing efforts.

Several studies have shown a direct correlation between employee job satisfaction and increased customer satisfaction and profits.

In an article appearing in *The Wall Street Journal*, Shellenbarger (1998, p. B1) reported, "A growing number of employers suspect improving employee satisfaction will have an indirect but important effect on profit. Some are running mountains of data through elaborate computer models to measure the links between employee satisfaction, customer satisfaction and revenue. The trend has major implications for people's ability to balance work with family and personal life."

According to Shellenbarger, Sears Roebuck conducted a study in 800 stores that measured employees' attitudes about their workload, treatment by bosses, and eight other human resource factors. The study found that those factors had a measurable effect on customer satisfaction and revenue. The conclusion was that a happy employee would continue employment with the company, give better service to customers, and recommend company products to others. Sears found that if employee attitudes on ten essential factors improved by just 5 percent, customer satisfaction jumped 1.3 percent, driving a one-half percent rise in revenue.

Shellenbarger also reported that Northern Telecom of Toronto was able to establish "conclusive evidence that improving employee satisfaction will satisfy customers better and, in turn, improve financial results." Also, Electronic Data Systems found that "employee-satisfaction data help predict costly turnover" (p. B1).

An in-depth study by the Gallup Organization identified twelve worker beliefs that play the biggest role in triggering a profitable, productive workplace. The Society for Human Resource Management reported that "analysis showed a consistent, reliable relationship between the 12 beliefs and the bottom line, such as profits, productivity, employee retention and customer loyalty. Organizations whose support of the statements ranked in the top 25 percent averaged 24 percent higher profitability, 29 percent higher revenue and 10 percent lower employee turnover than business units which scored lowest on the statements" (Micco, 1998, p. 16).

Not everyone accepts the theory that organizations should create positive work environments in order to increase employee satisfaction. There are those who believe that employers have no obligation to provide anything other than a fair wage for a decent day's work. Others believe this interest in positive work environments is a sign of a declining work ethic.

However, Thurow (1985, p. 142) makes this point: "The desire to make work self-fulfilling, less dangerous, cleaner, and more pleasant is not evidence of a declining work ethic. Given that Americans spend an enormous portion of their life on the job, it is natural that they wish to have a pleasant environment at work. Americans can work just as hard at a self-fulfilling, safe, clean, pleasant job as they do at a boring, dangerous, dirty, unpleasant job."

Thurow drew the conclusion from his research that as Americans spend more time on the job and less time with family, friends, neighbors, and church, they expect their workplace to provide a substitute for the satisfactions they used to get elsewhere. "Widespread demands for more meaningful work are not surprising. People want to work, but what they expect from work has changed just as they have changed" (p. 142).

Naisbitt and Aburdene (1985, p. 12) write, "The new re-invented corporations stress inordinate regard for the two most important types of people in an enterprise: employees and customers. They have discovered that by being both pro-people and pro-profits, a company can earn more than if it had targeted profits as its only goal. . . . It is not a question of being nice to people. It is simply a recognition that human beings will make or break a company."

Shellenbarger (1998, p. B1) quoted Robert Kaplan, a Harvard Business School accounting professor and coauthor of *The Balanced Scorecard*, who compared employer sensitivity on balancing work and personal life with corporate quality initiatives: "If you're out of control on it [balancing work and personal life], it's going to hurt performance. Then, you don't even get a chance to implement your [corporate] strategy because key people leave."

Characteristics of Positive Work Environments

Many people describe a good employer more easily by what it is not than by what it is. We may know it when we see it, but we have a hard time defining it.

One reason we have difficulty explaining why one employer is better than another, according to Levering (1988, pp. 18–19), is due "to the lack of a conceptual framework that lets us see how various policies and practices relate to each other. We don't understand the underlying principles of the workplace. The absence of concepts to appraise companies as workplaces contrasts with the abundance of tools to assess companies as businesses." We use market share to explain how well a company is doing relative to its competitors. We use sales growth to explain company growth. We use stock prices for for-profit corporations. And we use margin as a basic barometer of a health care organization's financial health. There are few consistent measurement tools for companies as workplaces. With financial performance, Levering said, we are not limited to saying that a company is doing well or doing poorly and giving some random facts or anecdotes to support our opinion.

But characteristics that are common to positive work environments are beginning to be defined through a variety of research projects. Positive work environments are not merely policies and procedures that can be duplicated exactly from workplace to workplace. In fact, Levering wrote that "at good workplaces, the whole is greater than the sum of its policies and procedures." He asserts that if "companies are good workplaces, it is not because of any specific policies. Far more important than the specific policies is the nature of the relationship between the company and the employees" (pp. 21–22).

There have been various surveys of job factors that are important to employees, compared with how supervisors and managers rate factors important to employees. In general, managers rate salary and benefits much higher than employees do. Employees tend to rate such factors as meaningful work, respectful treatment of employees by management, and genuine appreciation for employees' work as more important.

The soft factors of relationships are more important to employees than the hard factors of salaries, benefits, and policies. Health care administrators need to begin to pay more attention to these soft factors. For instance, an organization seeking to understand the reasons for high employee turnover may need to look more closely at the characteristics of the employment relationship rather than whether former employees were or were not pleased with benefits.

Levering (1988, p. 26) describes three important relationships: the relationship between the company and the employee, the relationship between the employee and the supervisor, and relationships among employees. He summarizes, "from an employee viewpoint, a great workplace is one in which you trust the people you work for, have pride in what you do, and enjoy the people you are working with."

In his book *A Journey into the Heroic Environment*, Lebow (1990) outlined the "Eight Principles of the Heroic Environment," which parallel the findings of Levering and Thurow. The principles are:

1. Treat others with uncompromising truth.
2. Lavish trust on your associates.
3. Mentor unselfishly.
4. Be receptive to new ideas regardless of their origin.
5. Take personal risks for the organization's sake.
6. Give credit where it's due.
7. Do not touch dishonest dollars.
8. Put the interests of others before your own (p. 19).

Lebow lists five steps toward heroic behavior:

1. Give and receive permission to act with autonomy.
2. Treat others as significant.
3. Make everyone feel like an insider.
4. Trust.
5. Act with integrity (p. 55).

Merely stating such principles or values is not enough. Follow-through is vital. For example, many companies have written values statements that do not accurately reflect the actions that managers take on a day-to-day basis. Stockholders, stakeholders, board members, and customers must make sure that senior management is aware of how policies, procedures, and actions support or defeat the stated values. Matejka (1991, pp. 17–18) wrote that one reason values are not always carried through is that "as top management changes, so do the values that are the driving force behind corporate priorities and goals. Most middle managers, when asked to write down the mission, values, and goals of their corporation, have great difficulty naming them. How can employees all move in the same direction when their managers cannot even clearly state that direction? Clarity is job 1! Commitment is job 2! Quality is job 3! Our corporations have lost their identity, and their clarity. Corporate amnesia has contributed greatly to the loss of competitive advantage."

Changes in mission, vision, and values that occur with a new chief executive, or to a lesser extent with newcomers to the organization in other management positions, can be lessened when an organization promotes from within. Employees who work their way up in the organization become familiar with the organization's mission, vision, and values and by nature of their continued employment have bought into the vision (unless negative rewards are in place). This consistency in mission, vision, and values can be seen in world-class organizations such as those profiled in books such as *The Leadership Moment* (Useem, 1998) and *Built to Last: Successful Habits of Visionary Companies* (Collins and Porras, 1995).

Improved financial performance is the by-product of a positive work environment, not a goal with which to attempt to motivate employees. Thurow (1985) said the knee-jerk reaction of motivating employees is not the answer.

> Motivation, cooperation, and teamwork are not a matter of persuasion or company pep talks or even of better managers. Lip service in praise of quality-control circles without actual shared decision making won't work. If the corporate goal remains the traditional maximization of shareholders' net worth, there will be no fundamental improvements in soft productivity. Firms cannot fool even half of

their workers even half of the time. Workers know when corporate goals are congruent with their own long-run self-interest and when they are not [p. 160].

Vroom (1964, p. 266) concluded that "workers perform most effectively when performance is a means of attaining goals which are extrinsic to the content of the work. We observed that the level of performance of workers is related to the extent to which performance is instrumental to the attainment of higher wages, promotions, and acceptance by co-workers. In each case this relationship is strongest for workers who most strongly value each of these outcomes."

The commitment and loyalty that employers are trying to encourage in their workforce is not merely a "touchy-feely" psychological ploy. Says Levering (1988, p. 6), "Within an organization, this feeling (of being a family) does more than engender camaraderie. It also helps the organization achieve its goals more effectively. This is one factor that explains why good employers tend to be more productive and profitable than their competitors."

Obstacles to Creating Positive Work Environments

A recent cartoon ("Bizarro" by Dan Piraro) showed a man lying on a psychiatrist's couch. The patient says to the doctor, "A year ago, I answered an ad that said 'Be Your Own Boss.' Now I can't help but see myself as a stupid, arrogant jackass who's trying to make my life miserable." Cartoons such as this one and "Dilbert" constantly ridicule the absurdity so many of us find in our work environments. Even the title of Levering's book (1988), *A Great Place to Work: What Makes Some Employers So Good (And Most So Bad)*, is an example of the rarity of positive work environments.

If we can show a positive correlation between organizational performance and positive work environments and if we can identify characteristics of positive work environments, why are there so few of them?

One explanation is the fundamental reason for being in business: to make a profit by providing a valued product or service. We can also look back to Levering's assertion that we have the tools to measure financial productivity and not work environments. Another answer from Lebow (1990, p. 16) says that "most work environments, instead of fostering unselfish behavior, discourage it."

Another factor is how the majority of senior executives in health care have been taught. Most master's programs, whether in health care administration or business, spend considerably more time on financial matters than on human resource administration, psychology, or organizational development. In fact, most of the latter courses are offered as electives rather than required courses. Most health care administrators have been well schooled in the hard factors and not so well instructed in the soft factors, which, ironically, are inherently more difficult to deal with.

According to Thurow (1985, p. 151): "The charge is also made that American industry has too many new MBAs who are taught that the short-run bottom line is the only thing . . . that it is easier to teach the quantitative methods that are applicable in short-run profit maximization where most of the parameters of the problem are known, than it is to teach long-run profit maximization where risk, uncertainty, and the unknown dominate."

According to Thurow, the fundamental goals of managers and workers are in direct opposition to each other. He says future executives are taught in school

> that the corporation exists *solely* to maximize the net worth of stockholder equity. The stock market places the right net present value on the future stream of profits, and it is the job of the shareholders' agents, the managers, to maximize that stock market value. In this model the absentee owners are wealth maximizers—nothing more, nothing less. Similarly, employees wish to maximize the net present value of their earnings—nothing more, nothing less. The owners of a corporation and its employees are natural adversaries. Workers want to maximize wages and minimize profits.

Owners and managers want to maximize profits and minimize wages
[p. 157].

Thurow (pp. 143–144) quotes a study conducted by Daniel
Yankelovich and John Immerwarh entitled "Putting the Work
Ethic to Work." This study found through public opinion polls that
"only 24 percent of the work force say that they are performing to
their full capacity ('being as effective as they are capable of
being')," yet 82 percent say they are interested in improving their
effectiveness. They believe there is a large gap between what they
are doing and what they could be doing—which suggests a major
source of productivity improvement.

The study reported that workers want greater autonomy, challenge, and interpersonal contact. Eighty percent reported they would
do a better job if they were more involved in decisions relating to their
work. Twenty-six percent said they want to develop themselves as
persons compared with only 10 percent of their parents.

Thurow concluded from the study that the American workforce wants to work, produce a high-quality product, and be
involved in making products and jobs better. However, society has
a workforce that is often unproductive, uninvolved, and produces
a low-quality product at what it regards as a low-quality job. He
concludes, "reducing the gap between these high aspirations and
the reality of a poor performance has to be the major task of American management" (p. 143). He believes that it is the employer's
responsibility to help employees be more productive by creating a
workforce that can work together as a team to raise productivity.
"America's biggest handicap is found in its inability to generate an
environment where the labor force takes a direct interest in raising
productivity. A high-quality well-motivated workforce interested
in working together as a team to raise productivity is ultimately the
major source of productivity growth" (pp. 148–149, referring to
Simmons and Mares, *Working Together*, New York: Knopf, 1983).

The recent Gallup Organization survey mentioned earlier
showed that individual managers make more of a difference in

employee satisfaction and productivity than the organization's policies. According to a review printed in *The Economist* ("It's the Manager, Stupid" 1998), the survey studied more than 100,000 employees in several hundred individual units of twenty-four large companies over twenty-five years. The survey's conclusion was that individual managers are important to unit success. The business units where employees were the happiest were often the most successful. Individual managers matter because the survey measured employee satisfaction "in terms of things that are controlled by individual managers, such as clear performance targets, the availability of proper equipment for a job, the presence of competent colleagues, and the attention of a caring supervisor." One reason that good practices do not spread within firms is that "managers often fear that borrowing ideas from their colleagues will boost the latter's status, at their own expense" (p. 54).

It would appear that incongruity between stated values and actions, traditional management education, and internal politics are among the reasons that positive work environments are not more common.

Conclusion: Moving Beyond the Common

In order to move beyond the common unfulfilling employment experience, health care organizations can look to two seemingly unrelated yet very similar departments. The human resources department and the marketing department both speak as the conscience of the organization representing employees and the public when organizational policies and special interests are contradictory. As advocates for these two constituencies, they need to be meaningful partners in the inner circle of senior management, and they need to see each other as allies, not adversaries as is so often the case.

In this book, we define the functions and responsibilities of the two departments more broadly than many in the health care industry and we will go into more detail throughout the book. For now, let us define them by their various titles within organizations. *Marketing* includes community relations, business development, corporate communications, public relations, community relations, planning and marketing, strategic planning, and marketing communications functions. *Human resources* includes personnel, organizational development, and education and training functions.

In the interest of clarity and understanding we also need to define *health care organizations* and *employees,* terms we will use throughout this book. The business of health care, ultimately, is patient care. Therefore, when we refer to *health care organizations* we are talking about any organization that provides, facilitates, or allows for the provision of care to patients. This can mean hospitals, integrated delivery systems, surgery centers, immediate care centers, long-term care facilities, nursing homes, assisted living centers, managed care organizations, physician offices, insurance companies, alternative care providers, or any other organization that provides health care. But we always refer to *health care organizations* in the context of patients.

It is important to recognize that there are times when the term *employees* not only includes persons actually employed by an institution, but also the physicians and volunteers who provide direct service to patients. Physicians and volunteers have to be just as attuned to customer service issues as traditionally defined employees. Many patients have difficulty understanding the relationships between physicians, hospitals, insurance companies, and other providers. In fact, many consumers assume all physicians are employed by hospitals and have difficulty understanding any kind of adversarial relationship between health care providers and physicians.

Organizations that recognize the importance of linking their performance measurements to strategy are in a position to maximize returns, improve quality outcomes, and increase their value in the community. The benefits of linking human resources and marketing functions in your organization include

- *Easier recruiting*. You will experience fewer voluntary terminations and will receive more qualified applications for open positions, resulting in less expense to the organization.

- *Reduced turnover and absenteeism rates*. Employees who are appropriately recruited and trained and who receive appropriate incentives to remain with the organization are more satisfied and less likely to voluntarily terminate employment, take inappropriate sick days, or become sick due to stress-induced illnesses. Unfortunately, since many health care organizations currently do not track turnover and absentee rates, or know the cost of these to the organization, it will be difficult to measure improvements in this area.

- *Lower marketing expense*. When your employees market your services through their high-quality performance, you have less dissonance to overcome in the market, therefore less promotional expense. However, to improve employee performance, money from promotional budgets may have to be allocated to other line items such as market research, physical plant renovations, computer systems, and so on.

- *Greater profitability*. By reducing expenses in recruitment and marketing and decreasing voluntary turnover and inappropriate absenteeism, the organization's expenses can be drastically reduced.

This new linkage will cause you to challenge some fundamental premises of your organization. The willingness to pursue new ways of doing business requires not only leadership in an intellectual sense, but also courage and risk taking. It requires a willingness to let go of familiar patterns and behavior and seek new ways of doing things, even if they are difficult, uncomfortable, and unfamiliar.

We ask you to think beyond yourself to the best outcome for your organization, its employees, your community, and your patients. Some recent health care management advice read, "Your career survival is primary." We disagree. Patient care is primary. Through the achievement of organizational goals that improve the quality of life of your patients and community, your career survival will take care of itself.

Case Study:
An Employer of Choice, Eli Lilly and Company

In every community, there is one employer who develops and maintains a reputation as "the place to work." Whether large or small, even children know that's where they'd like to work when they grow up. Not only does the company pay well, but it treats its people fairly. "If you can get in, you're set," people are heard to say.

In the Indianapolis metropolitan area, that employer has been Eli Lilly and Company.* But the company's reputation is growing nationally and internationally as well because of a variety of programs that foster respect for employees and their families. Maintaining that "employer-of-choice" reputation for generations is a difficult and admirable thing to do.

Lilly "started as a family business, and it has always been known as a good employer," said Candice Lange, director, Human Resources, Workforce Partnering Initiatives. "Even during the Depression, there were never any layoffs. Employees may have had to cut the grass if there was nothing else to do, but they kept their jobs."

The new workforce that began emerging in the 1980s provided new challenges to the company to maintain their status. "People needed something different from the workplace," said Lange. "We surveyed employees and found that only 18 percent were part of a traditional family structure that included the man working and the woman staying at home taking care of children. A significant number of our workers were single, and many of them had children to care for. That was when we started looking at work–[personal] life balance issues. This is where a lot of our flexible scheduling came from. The three main issues we were looking at were dependent care, flex time, and management awareness of work–[personal] life issues."

---

*This case study is based on an interview with Candice Lange, director, Human Resources, Workforce Partnering Initiatives, Eli Lilly and Company, Indianapolis, November 23, 1998.

According to Lange, Lilly recognizes the importance of helping employees with their work and personal issues because it realized that "people bring their entire selves to work. We believe work should be fulfilling, not draining. Generation X workers often come from environments with little family support. The old policies and procedures don't make sense to them. We had to look at flexible starting and ending times for shifts to better adjust to their lifestyle."

Lange says Lilly has found that changes in policies at work have an impact on an individual employee's need to balance work and personal life.

> I've never heard anyone here say, "I wish I had an easier job." People like to be challenged. A lot of stress in the workplace is caused by lack of control. Flex policies are not as much about time as they are about control. If employees are worried about whether their kids get on the bus on time, they won't be concentrating on work. We went to the employees to find out how to define flex policies. We are always looking for a win-win situation. The key is to trust employees, get out of their way, and let them do their best work. Giving employees more control also contributes to an increase in teamwork. They depend on each other to help each other out.

The company's plans to maintain their employer-of-choice reputation in the future include continually surveying employees "to make sure we understand how the work is done from their perspective. There has been a nationwide shift in work philosophy due to Generation X. Many older workers are burned out because their family life isn't good. It's difficult to have a good work life if you don't have a good family life, and vice versa. There is a correlation between employee satisfaction and customer satisfaction. The way your internal customers look reflects the way your external customers see your company."

References

Collins, J. C., and Porras, J. I. *Built to Last: Successful Habits of Visionary Companies*. New York: HarperCollins, 1995.

"It's the Manager, Stupid." *The Economist*, Aug. 8, 1998.

Lebow, R. *A Journey into the Heroic Environment*. Rocklin, Calif.: Prima, 1990.

Levering, R. *A Great Place to Work: What Makes Some Employers So Good (And Most So Bad)*. New York: Random House, 1988.

Matejka, K. *Why This Horse Won't Drink: How to Win—and Keep—Employee Commitment*. New York: AMACOM, 1991.

Mathis, R. L., and Jackson, J. H. *Human Resource Management*. (8th ed.) St. Paul, Minn.: West, 1997.

Micco, L. "Gallup Study Links Worker Beliefs, Increased Productivity." *HRNews*, Society for Human Resource Management, Sept. 1998.

Mycek, S. "Leadership for a Healthy 21st Century." *Healthcare Forum Journal*, July/Aug. 1998.

Naisbitt, J., and Aburdene, P. *Re-inventing the Corporation*. New York: Warner Books, 1985.

Shellenbarger, S. "Work and Family: Companies Are Finding It Really Pays to Be Nice to Employees." *The Wall Street Journal*, July 22, 1998.

Thurow, L. C. *The Zero-Sum Solution: Building a World Class American Economy*. New York: Simon & Schuster, 1985.

Useem, M. *The Leadership Moment*. New York: Times Business/Random House, 1998.

Vroom, V. *Work and Motivation*. New York: Wiley, 1964.

Chapter Two

Creating and Evaluating
Mission, Vision, and Values

The purpose of mission, vision, and values statements is to focus an organization on what is important, how to meet customers' needs, and how to help employees fulfill the organization's goals. From a practical standpoint, the statements provide common definitions that drive strategy, goals, and objectives—but only when daily decisions are based on the statements.

Mission, vision, and values are sometimes viewed differently at different levels of the organization. Whereas senior and middle-level managers may be proponents of formal statements, front-line employees may question the need for such formalities, especially when organizational practice conflicts with written statements. An individual employee's perspective significantly affects his or her willingness to embrace the various components of the statements and work toward achieving the organization's goals.

It is important to remember that even if your organization does not have formal mission, vision, and values statements, an informal understanding of culture, goals, and acceptable behavior does exist. However, the lack of written statements leads to confusion among employees and between employees and managers. When employees do not have a clear understanding of goals, they make well-intentioned decisions that they believe are correct but that may be, in fact, in direct opposition to company goals and in conflict with other decisions being made within the company. Likewise, there is a great deal of effort expended by employees in such companies in discussing or arguing the appropriate decision to be made for a particular situation.

Formal statements can help an organization achieve its goals only if the statements are clear, concise, communicated, and carried out. With a clear definition of what you do and where you are going, you—and more important, your employees—will know how to recognize when goals are achieved and which decisions must be made along the way.

In this chapter, we will provide an overview of the distinctions between mission, vision, and values, describe the key elements of each, and discuss how to develop and evaluate mission, vision, and values statements.

Distinctions Between Mission, Vision, and Values

Not all organizations will have all three types of statements. Health care organizations may incorporate their values into their mission statement, have one statement that encompasses all three aspects, or make the mission, vision, and values statements three distinct documents. For the sake of a common understanding, we define the three statements as:

- *Mission: the current reality.* This is your core purpose—what you are, what you do, the reason you are in business.
- *Vision: the dream.* This is the statement of what you want to be or what you want to create within your organization or community.
- *Values: organizational ethics.* These are the principles of right and wrong in behavior—what your organization stands for and the kind of behavior it expects its employees to exhibit. In essence, established values create a corporate code of conduct.

Mission

Your organization's mission statement describes who you are and what you do. The mission is the operational, ethical, and financial guideline of the company. Through your mission, you articulate the purpose, goals, behavior, culture, and strategies of your organization. The mission provides a constancy of purpose for everyone within the organization to embrace and understand. It includes the core purpose of the organization—those things that will not change over time.

A health care organization that intends to succeed in the future cannot be all things to all people. Although both ends of the health care spectrum serve a necessary purpose, one hospital cannot be both a large, high-tech tertiary care center and a small, primary care community hospital. A clearly defined mission statement eliminates conflicts within the organization by allowing clearer decision making. When decisions are based on a clear, concise, and mutually agreed on mission statement, everyone in the organization can work from the same page.

The following are the key elements of a mission statement:

- Identify who you are.
- Describe what you do.
- Determine for whom you do it.
- Explain the core business purpose.

The process you choose to craft a mission statement will depend on a variety of factors, including your organization's culture. Some mission statements are developed from the top down, with the CEO or other senior managers drafting a statement and then seeking input from others within the organization. Other statements are written from the bottom up, with significant input and word crafting from front-line staff before the final approval is given by senior management and the board. Whichever way your organization has drafted, or intends to draft, its mission statement, you may want to review the mission statements of other organizations.

One excellent resource is a book by Jones and Kahaner (1995), *Say It and Live It: 50 Corporate Mission Statements That Hit the Mark*.

This book includes the mission statements for fifty U.S. companies, along with a brief discussion of each. They found "successful, exciting, and powerful companies that had true values. Their mission statements were not just concepts and philosophies they had cobbled together but were well-thought-out ideas that had helped them meet and exceed their financial dreams, treat their employees well, break free of a crisis, and stake out a piece of 'the right thing to do.' They were road maps for the high road" (p. x).

Each organization's mission statement is going to be different, reflecting the unique aspects of its core purpose, services, and customers. But there are common characteristics that can be useful in preparing a mission statement or evaluating an existing one. We suggest using the guidelines in Figure 2.1.

The mission statement should be evaluated at least annually by employees, management, and the board using the criteria in Figure 2.1. Word crafting should be avoided; changing a "would" to a "should" or adding or deleting a word here or there is not the issue in evaluation. The critical issue is whether or not the mission statement accurately reflects the organization's core purpose: what it does and for whom. Only when there is a discrepancy between the reality and the mission statement should it be changed.

Vision

If the mission defines the current state and purpose of the organization, the vision describes its hopes and dreams. A clear vision is necessary in order to effect change within an organization or community. Because of the speed and intensity of change within society in general and health care in particular, creating and communicating a shared vision helps ensure that all members of the organization are working toward the same goal.

A vision is a picture of how things could be, how you want them to be, and how you can make the current situation better. Creating a vision builds expectations that something will change.

Figure 2.1. Mission Statement Guidelines.

The following are guidelines for health care organizations to create and evaluate mission statements.

- *Keep it simple*. Explain what you do and for whom. The mission explains your organization's core reason for existence. It should be easily understood by everyone in the organization and everyone you serve.

- *Allow input*. It does not matter whether the mission statement starts from the top down or bottom up, there should be substantial opportunities for individuals from all levels and areas of the organization to provide input so that everyone agrees that the mission statement accurately reflects the organization's purpose.

- *Bring in fresh perspectives*. Persons outside the organization can often bring clarity and a fresh perspective to the creation or evaluation of your mission statement. This could include a professional consultant, but could also be members of your community, your patients, or other key stakeholders. You and your employees know your organization best, but someone outside the company can provide valuable input. Outside input is also extremely important to assess the disharmony between perceived and internal and external realities. Your current mission may have changed significantly from its original mission, which is still perceived by your community as the reason you exist.

- *Be believable*. The wording and tone should reflect your personality or what you would like your personality to be. Pretentious wording would be inconsistent with a simple philosophy and viewed as unnatural. Use words that your audience will understand. Just because a mission statement is important to the organization's ability to meet its goals does not mean that it has to be difficult to understand.

- *Communicate*. Share the mission statement in as many ways as possible and in as many languages as necessary. Highlight key words or rephrase the core statement into simpler language. Keep the mission in front of people constantly through the use of wallet cards, framed copies in offices and public areas, as screen savers, and as a standard agenda item for regular staff meetings, strategy meetings, and retreats.

- *Live it*. Rely on the mission statement for guidance. Challenge it continuously by asking yourself on a regular basis whether this mission still fits. The mission statement should not only be written, it should be lived. You should judge your own actions and those of fellow employees by how well you and they adhere to its principles.

Source: Adapted from Jones and Kahaner, 1995, pp. 263–267.

A vision creates a sense of urgency and explains where the organization wants to go, why it needs to change, and the broad parameters of how it will get to the new reality. A vision statement, like a mission statement, must be written in simple, natural language. You should be able to describe your vision in less than five minutes. If you can't explain your vision in two or three sentences and receive feedback that the vision is understandable, you do not have a clearly defined vision.

The following are the key elements of a vision statement:

- Incorporate a sense of urgency in the wording.
- Determine where you are going.
- Explain why you are going there.
- Use simple, natural language.

In a small organization of one to twenty employees, it is easy to create and communicate the vision. In a larger organization with its inherent communication challenges, it is necessary to develop a clear, concise vision in order to bring all employees together so everyone can see where they are going. A clear vision is needed so life tomorrow can be made better than it is today or to ensure continued success for the organization.

Characteristics of the Vision. In addition to the key elements, a vision has the following characteristics that will help your organization develop or evaluate your vision:

- *It is appropriate.* The vision is right for the community, the organization, and its customers and employees. The vision fits the current or future environment and is appropriate to the company's mission.
- *It is achievable.* The vision should include energetic goals that the organization is capable of achieving. The vision should stretch the organization's capabilities, but not to the breaking

point. The goal should be high, yet realistic and attainable. It is also important to pay attention to the competencies and individual abilities necessary to realize the vision. These abilities must be identified and fostered throughout the process of achieving the goal. Setting a vision without doing what is necessary to help employees achieve it is a prescription for failure, disappointment, disenchantment, and turnover.

- *It clarifies.* An effective vision provides direction, guidance, and structure to the organization. It allows employees to be able to make daily decisions without constant direction from supervisors and senior management. Too often change is perceived by employees as something that is being taken away. It is important, therefore, to make sure that the vision does not take something away without replacing it with something at least as good or better and that it is communicated well. An effective vision provides something all employees can work toward because it will be different and better than what exists today.

- *It is conveyable.* A clear and effective vision is easy to communicate. It is not just senior management who need to communicate the vision. All employees should be able to explain the vision to someone outside the organization within five minutes and receive feedback that it was easily understood. The most effective vision statements are written in simple, natural language.

- *It is credible.* An effective vision paints a believable picture of what the future will look like. Everyone within the organization believes that the vision is both appropriate and possible for the group together to accomplish. Employees believe that the vision is achievable for this particular organization and that it is necessary to accomplish it for future success.

- *It is desirable.* The vision appeals to the long-term interests of employees, customers, stockholders, and others who have a stake in the enterprise. The vision clearly organizes employees' perceptions. If they don't believe, they cannot see the improvements and therefore cannot act in a manner consistent with the vision. And if they do not see or agree with the vision, they may not be appropriate employees for that organization. The vision must resonate with those involved in implementing it.

- *It differentiates the organization from others.* The purpose of a vision is to create change and focus employees' energies on improving the current state of the organization. Within that, a vision involves superlatives or unique achievements that differentiate your organization from others. An effective vision should distinguish your organization from others in your industry or community.

- *It energizes.* A vision is motivating. It grabs attention, focuses and arouses passion, transforms purpose into action, compels employees, pulls people toward it, commits people to action, drives a stake in the ground, says "that's what we will be." It becomes a rallying point for people inside and outside the organization (Boylan, 1995, p. 51). A vision is inspirational in that it provides an opportunity for employees to be involved in something larger than themselves and contribute to a larger society and achievement.

- *It is flexible.* An effective vision is general enough to allow individual initiative and alternative responses depending on the changing environment. It enables flexibility in executing the specific details that will achieve the larger goal. The vision establishes parameters within which each employee may act to accomplish it.

- *It is focused.* A clear, focused vision provides guidance in decision making so that individual employees may act without constant supervision. According to Kotter (1996, pp. 7–8), "Vision plays a key role in producing useful change by helping to direct, align and inspire actions on the part of large numbers of people. Without an appropriate vision, a transformation effort can easily dissolve into a list of confusing, incompatible, and time-consuming projects that go in the wrong direction or nowhere at all. Without a vision to guide decision making, each and every choice employees face can dissolve into an interminable debate. The smallest of decisions can generate heated conflict that saps energy and destroys morale." Without an effective vision that provides clear direction, chaos would prevail, as it does in many organizations undergoing change.

- *It predicts future actions.* As futurist Leland Kaiser has explained on many occasions, once a mind has embraced a new idea, it begins creating that vision. Kotter (1996, pp. 68–69) writes:

  Vision refers to a picture of the future with some implicit or explicit commentary on why people should strive to create that future. In a change process, a good vision serves three important purposes. First, by clarifying the general direction for change, by saying the corporate equivalent of "we need to be south of here in a few years instead where we are today," it simplifies hundreds or thousands of more detailed decisions. Second, it motivates people to take action in the right direction, even if the initial steps are personally painful. Third, it helps coordinate the actions of different people, even thousands and thousands of individuals, in a remarkably fast and efficient way.

- *It conveys a sense of urgency.* A compelling vision explains to an organization's stakeholders where the organization needs to go and why. Particularly when an organization has been successful, it may be difficult for employees to understand why change is necessary to remain competitive in the future. A successful vision provides enough detail for all concerned to understand and embrace the vision—or choose to leave the organization if the vision does not correspond with their beliefs.

- *It is time specific.* A vision must have a time-specific goal to work toward. Gauging success in achieving a goal requires a time period by which to measure.

Creating a Vision. As with a mission statement, the process of creating a vision must fit with the organization's needs and culture. Because front-line employees are not aware of all the trends within an industry and are generally more operationally than strategically focused, the creation of the vision usually rests with senior management and the board. But employee input should be sought, seriously considered, and incorporated.

Creating a vision requires a truthful internal and external assessment, gathering information and input from throughout the organization, a bit of organizational soul searching, and a continuous commitment to clarify, reassess, and readjust the vision every year.

Futurist Leland Kaiser (1995) has written and lectured to thousands of health care leaders on the process of vision. Kaiser believes firmly in the power of thought: that an individual or an organization can create an alternative future by discussing the possibilities and then identifying reachable futures. According to Kaiser, "when you think it, it's real." The question then becomes, how do you fund, staff, and create that vision? The prevailing mind-set of the institution determines its future. When you create the appropriate conditions or circumstances, manifestation occurs; action today frames the future.

Kaiser agrees with Stephen Covey that you must begin with the end in mind. "The best designers design from end to beginning. Describe the destination. Where are you now? How to get from here to there? You can change your future as quickly as you change your mind."

To create the vision, you must think in terms of the future and ask yourselves the following series of questions:

- What is likely to occur in the next three, five, ten years?
- What will happen to your organization in that time if you do nothing different from what you are doing today?
- What is the best thing you can imagine happening?

- What is the preferred situation for your organization?
- What is a realistic, achievable vision to accomplish in three, five, ten years?

Kaiser recommends two methods for creating a vision:

Assumption reversal. Take the prevailing assumptions and turn them around. According to Kaiser, an assumption is an excuse not to do something. For instance, many health care organizations over the past decade have reversed the assumption that patients come to the hospital. Hundreds of clinics have been established in community centers, churches, schools, and rural areas as a result of this assumption reversal.

Constraint removal. Several methods of constraint removal are possible, including:

- *Best of all worlds.* Create your ideal picture of what the best possible world would look like and how your organization would fit into that world.
- *Starting over with a blank sheet.* Pretend that the health care industry did not exist. How would you structure it? What would it look like? Who would provide the care? For whom?
- *Creating new metaphors.* Look at your organization from the standpoint of a different industry. What would your organization be like if it were operated as a bank, a school, an amusement park, a restaurant?
- *That which could never happen.* Be outrageous and ridiculous in your predictions of the future.
- *Guided fantasy.* Think of the most futuristic system imaginable.
- *Taking the standpoint of another.* Look at your organization from the perspective of your patients, medical staff, volunteers, visitors, and employees. How would they recreate your organization to fit their needs better?

Kaiser's steps to create a vision listed in Figure 2.2 include both individual and group vision processes.

Some companies have been so successful over a long period that they can be called visionary companies. In most cases, these companies did not have traditionally defined visionary leaders, but each employee within the organization steadfastly held to the well-defined and adhered-to mission, vision, and values in achieving company goals. These companies were profiled in the book *Built to Last* by Collins and Porras (1995), who found that visionary companies create and nurture a set of core values and a purpose that do not change, and they are eternally vigilant to the creation of alignment between the vision and action.

As with any enterprise, there will be obstacles in the implementation of the vision. The corporate culture, organizational structure, management practices, and reward systems must align with the vision.

Figure 2.2. Steps in the Vision Creation Process.

- Generate images.
- Identify with the image.
- Gain group consensus of the vision.
- Desire the vision to become reality and will that the vision will occur.
- Permeate the organization with the vision and act to begin implementing it.
- Work through the counterreaction to the vision (resistance to change).
- Add density (pictures, images, stories) to the vision.
- Act as a channel for manifestation of the vision and make adjustments as necessary (changing situations, regulations, and so on).
- Enjoy the realization of your vision and realize that at some point you have to let go of the vision.
- Take what you have learned and generate a new and more powerful vision.
- Repeat the creation process.

Source: Kaiser, 1995.

Kotter (1996, p. 10) points out that among the obstacles are organizational structure, narrow job descriptions, compensation and performance appraisal systems that require people to choose between change and self-interest, and persons (particularly managers) who are invested in the old system and refuse to change.

It is extremely difficult for people who created a culture to change it. We are all resistant to change to some degree. But individuals within an organization who have the most to gain by the maintenance of the status quo can be damaging to the achievement of the vision and employee morale. When a vision that is highly desired by everyone but a few within the organization is allowed to be undermined by those few, management credibility is damaged unless they are dealt with in a firm manner. "Whenever smart and well-intentioned people avoid confronting obstacles, they disempower employees and undermine change," writes Kotter (1996, p. 11).

The vision and the changes it will create must be anchored in the corporate culture, according to Kotter. "Until new behaviors are rooted in social norms and shared values, they are always subject to degradation as soon as the pressure associated with a change effort are removed" (p. 14).

Evaluating the Vision.   Once each year, senior management and the board should review the vision to make sure it remains meaningful and important. You should evaluate the vision according to the characteristics listed earlier in this chapter. Plus, you will want to ask these questions about your vision statement:

- What are the key words in the vision statement?
- How do you feel about the statement?
- Does it create a sense of personal identification? If not, how would it have to change for you to feel a sense of ownership?
- Is the vision meaningful to you? If not, how would it have to change to be meaningful? (Senge and others, 1994, p. 339)

Values

Whereas the mission statement defines what you do and the vision statement defines what you want to be in the future, your values define your corporate code of conduct. They tell everyone what you stand for. Some management specialists recommend that you first discuss and define the organization's values and then move on to the vision statement.

"Values drive organizations—everything you do is based on the basic values by which you live your life," according to Boylan (1995), author of *Get Everyone in Your Boat Rowing in the Same Direction: 5 Leadership Principles to Follow So Others Will Follow You.* Values shape:

- *Attitudes*—how you develop people
- *Policies*—how you treat personnel issues
- *Procedures*—how fast you do things or to what degree of accuracy and quality
- *Activities*—how, or if, you really celebrate victories (p. 36)

Whether or not you actually have formal written values, your employees and customers will be able to tell you what the demonstrated values of your organization are. According to Boylan:

Values are always being demonstrated. You cannot hide them or claim that you have a certain value and then act differently, or you'll be (correctly) labeled a hypocrite. Values create your organization's culture—how the place lives as an entity. You, as a potential leader, have values. You already know what's important to you. Therefore, you need to clearly state those values to others. Be laser clear. Be brief. Then, find out who agrees with you. Those who do will follow you. Those who don't, won't. And shouldn't. Once you get people to agree on a set of mutual values, business objectives will be more easily defined [pp. 36–37].

The organization's direction is based on what everyone agrees are the values. Values create an environment in which it is easy for people to understand what is expected, buy in or buy out, or agree or disagree with the direction.

The following are the key elements of a values statement:

- The values support mission and vision.
- They are consistent with individual actions.
- They are defined by means of discussion throughout the organization.

Discussion of values in order to achieve mutual definitions is critical within your organization. For instance, if one of your values is to provide excellent customer service, some employees may feel that the "golden rule" is a good measure of living that value. However, not all customers want to be treated the same way the employee providing the service does. Perhaps rather than treat others the way you want to be treated, you should treat others the way they want to be treated. This requires much more information about your customers individually and collectively and creates a very different customer service result. Without discussion about the definition of values, too much is left to chance.

Whether the values that the organization decides to espouse are right for everyone or not is not the issue. Things that some people value are not valued by others. The important thing is that the organization make a commitment to its values and create a consistent adherence to those values.

In fact, the authors of *Built to Last* found that one of the many myths about successful companies was that they shared a common subset of "correct" values.

[T]here is no "right" set of core values for beginning a visionary company. Indeed, two companies can have radically different ideologies, yet both be visionary. Core values in a visionary company don't even have to be "enlightened" or "humanistic," although they often are. The crucial variable is not the content of a company's ideology, but how deeply it believes its ideology and how consistently it lives, breathes and expresses it in all that it does. Visionary companies do not ask, "What should we value?" They ask "What do we actually value deep down to our toes?" [Collins and Porras, 1995, p. 8].

Regardless of the specific values your organization chooses to embrace, one value, whether stated or not, that each health care organization should espouse is integrity—in part because your patients expect it. Fulghum (1997, p. 75) defines this as *praxis*—activity as opposed to theory. "The older I get, the less attention I pay to what people say or think or hope. I notice what they do, how they live, and what they work for. There is an unresolved argument in the arts and in politics over whether one's words are to be judged with regard to one's life. I come down on the side of integrity: The life validates or invalidates the words."

Whitley and Heeley (1998, pp. 4–5) recommend a "culture of integrity," which can be achieved by a clear identity as defined by mission, values, and commitments, ongoing communication about the identity, and conduct consistent with the identity.

Senior leadership must start with trust, the underlying issue in leadership. Trust gets people on your side and keeps them there. To generate and sustain trust, leaders need:

- *Constancy*—whatever surprises leaders themselves may face, they should not create any for the group. Leaders must stay the course.

- *Congruity*—Leaders walk the talk. There is no gap between the theories they espouse and the life they practice.

- *Reliability*—Leaders are there when it counts, ready to support their team members as needed.

- *Integrity*—Leaders honor their commitments and promises (Cinergy Services, Inc., 1998, p. 29).

Conclusion

Together the mission, vision, and values define for employees, patients, medical staff, the community, and other stakeholders the core purpose of the organization, its beliefs, and its hopes and dreams. They also help employees make decisions on a daily basis of what to do, how to behave, and what their role in the future of the organization is. But written statements hung on a wall are useless unless they are effectively implemented. Implementation is the subject of the next chapter.

Case Study: A Vision-Driven Move at Methodist Hospital of Indiana, Inc.

In 1992, Martyn W. C. Howgill experienced one of those situations for which the phrase "be careful what you ask for because some day you might get it" was coined. Prior to joining Methodist Hospital of Indiana, Inc. (now one of three hospitals that make up Clarian Health Partners),* Howgill had spent five years at HCA Wesley in Kansas. "I had five years of intensive quality management training and embraced quality quite aggressively. I believe strongly in the principles of quality management and what marketing can accomplish." But with a background in journalism and communications, he was an unlikely candidate to add the human resources function to his responsibilities.

As senior vice president for marketing at Methodist, Howgill had been a frequent proponent of employee relations as it relates to a market-driven, customer service–oriented organization.

"I had been talking for some time in executive meetings about the need to treat employees in a certain way so they would

---

*This case study is based on interviews with Martyn W. C. Howgill, chief marketing officer, University of Texas, MD Anderson Cancer Center, Houston, October 19, 1998; and William Loveday, president and CEO, Clarian Health Partners, Indianapolis, February 16, 1999.

be customer service–oriented and we could be more market driven. We have customers of our processes. I believed that to get employees to think in those terms, we had to get HR involved," said Howgill.

The sudden death of the senior vice president for human resources presented an occasion for the organization to restructure its senior management team. "I had been rocking the boat about this," Howgill said, "so after Lee [Hansen] died, Bill came to me and said there were a lot of ways we could replace Lee, and one was that I could take the job. We kicked it around and decided 'let's give it a try.'" Howgill became senior vice president for human resources and marketing.

According to Bill Loveday, now president and CEO of Clarian Health Partners (then CEO at Methodist), the integration of the two departments was serendipitous. "What happened in our case is we had a fairly unique individual. It's somewhat unusual to have an executive with the skill set to manage two very distinct activities generally defined as marketing and human resources. Martyn was an early advocate of marketing's focus being on clinical quality, service excellence, quality improvement, not an advocate that marketing's job was advertising."

Among Howgill's reservations was that he did not have any background in human resources, although he had been a customer of HR and on occasion a dissatisfied one. Loveday's opinion was that there were many well-trained staff at the director level who had the technical knowledge; what they lacked was a vision for the organization and the culture necessary to deal with the rapid changes being presented by the marketplace. It seemed Howgill and Loveday were on the same page. Howgill states, "If we do a good job marketing and bring people to the organization and they have a bad experience, we're creating a problem by drawing attention to ourselves. Word of mouth is very effective, particularly with negative experience. So we focused on recruitment, training, customer orientation, and service sensitivity."

Loveday adds:

Anybody giving it any thought at all with a modern perspective on marketing would realize the natural linkage between hiring, training, retaining, measuring performance, and so forth as being an integral role and responsibility of marketing. Marketing is about results and taking a scientific approach; it's intimately concerned with the development of human capital in the organization and its performance. If that definition is focused broadly on customers, then it makes sense that there is a natural marriage of that effort with what human resources has been traditionally focused on. It requires a change in perspective of what human resources has traditionally been about and what modern marketing is about.

A number of projects went well according to Howgill. "We put together a vision of how we wanted to work together. We talked about this at the senior management level—how to treat one another with respect, trust one another, how we're all here to do the best job we can. We understood problems come from the variations (policies, tools, and so on—not people). We laid some initial groundwork."

Among the things the senior team looked at within the value system were pay structures. The previous evaluation process had linked annual performance evaluations with a merit pay system that provided some employees very small additional increases but was extremely divisive. Employees had to be in the "excellent" category for an employee to get a merit increase. The team determined there were problems with that system and abandoned it. They piloted different employee feedback methods and completely disconnected evaluations from compensation. For a given job, a pay range would be market competitive, recognizing that the market would vary geographically. There would be different quartiles for each job. The annual percentage increase would be the same across the board for every employee in the hospital. "Managers should be doing their job every day and providing support for people on a regular basis. Our position was that 'if you're here, by definition, you're doing a good job because our managers are regularly addressing those employees who need special assistance," Howgill said.

"While on occasion it may become necessary for an employee to leave, most of the time poor performance is because management hasn't provided the support or training an employee needs to do the job, or because a bad match has been made between the employee's skills and the job requirements. It is management's job to continually improve the screening, selection, and placement processes and then to support employees with their continuing requirements for training and education.

"This change had a significant impact on culture. There were some staff who did not like the change. When they complained about getting the same amount as the 'slackers' I asked them to identify those people. Of course, everybody thought it was other people who were not pulling their share of the load; it was never them. While there were some people who didn't like it, there were lots of positive comments—for example, 'for the first time, I am having a meaningful dialogue with my boss about my performance with no money involved in the conversation.' They had a more honest conversation," he said.

According to Howgill, changing the culture had its difficult times and it was hard to gain support quickly. A cost-cutting program accomplished through work redesign, called "Reinventing Methodist," was implemented in this same period, without layoffs. "It worked very well, but was quite disruptive," he said.

Employees—all of us—find it difficult to embrace change unless we understand what the future holds for us. But our commitment to treating each other with trust and respect and building a customer-driven culture forced us to focus not just on cutting out people as so many traditional lay-offs have done, but rather to redesign the work to require fewer people to do it. By eliminating the things that didn't add value for patients and their physicians and by reducing complexity and rework in the system, we were able to eliminate more than 600 "positions' worth" of work. Then we absorbed the staff in those positions by moving them into vacancies as they became available, by reducing overtime, and through a generous voluntary separation program. At the end, while nobody thought it was fun, I think most employees felt that management had done all it could to treat them fairly.

The decision to separate the two functions of marketing and human relations back into their traditional roles was made in 1996 when talks began between Indiana University Hospital (IU), Riley Hospital for Children, and Methodist Hospital to merge into Clarian Health Partners.

"It was apparent that IU had a totally different culture from Methodist and it was very clear to me that everything we had accomplished was going to be changed as a result. It would have been impossible to impose what we were doing on the IU culture," said Howgill. Because of concern on the part of IU that having a Methodist Hospital senior vice president oversee the creation of a new payroll, compensation, and benefits system for the new company would be perceived as a takeover by Methodist, Howgill chose to leave Methodist to become chief marketing officer of The University of Texas MD Anderson Cancer Center in Houston.

Howgill does not regret the attempt to align the two traditionally separate functions of HR and marketing. "If it's a stable organization and you have someone who has a clear vision of what the culture is and what it's supposed to do, it's a very good approach." He recommends good technical support if the manager is primarily familiar with one of the disciplines and the crucial understanding and support of the board and CEO.

Rather than looking at the structure of an integrated department, Loveday looks at the definitions of and working relationship between the two departments.

To me the question is not should they be under the same executive, it is: Is there a significant overlap between how people look at marketing today and its responsibilities? You can't argue for that [one

senior executive] as a way to go. You have to argue for the partnership—do they work together? You have to clarify roles and responsibilities, setting down the goals of HR and marketing. If your
approach to marketing is focused on performance—clinical, people, cost, service—if that's how you define marketing, the whole
issue of measurement, then you see the tremendous overlap
between the two. There are organizations that are not valuing marketing for the science it represents, organizations that do not have
marketing at a senior level. Marketing equals understanding the
customer and driving the organization to meet customer needs—
whether the customer is patient, family, physician, general public
or employee.

Health care organizations have traditionally undervalued and
underdefined marketing. The same is true with human resources,
being traditionally defined as cut-and-dried, detailed, bureaucratic,
function based, and limited to policies and procedures.

Human resources and marketing do not have to work together
every day, but the two departments need to continually identify
areas of overlap, Loveday said. "When you think of employees as
customers, it's vital to know what employees are thinking about.
The topic of employee satisfaction surveys often engenders a discussion about who's going to do the survey—marketing or human
resources. Both are capable of doing it and both need the information to do their jobs. Who cares who does it—they should be working together."

References

Boylan, B. *Get Everyone in Your Boat Rowing in the Same Direction: 5 Leadership
    Principles to Follow So Others Will Follow You*. Holbrook, Mass.: Adams
    Media, 1995.
Cinergy Services, Inc. *Building Healthy Communities*. Plainfield, Ind.: Cinergy
    Corporation, 1998.

Collins, J. C., and Porras, J. I. *Built to Last: Successful Habits of Visionary Companies*. New York: HarperCollins, 1995.

Fulghum, R. *Words I Wish I Wrote*. New York: HarperCollins, 1997.

Jones, P., and Kahaner, L. *Say It and Live It: 50 Corporate Mission Statements That Hit the Mark*. New York: Currency/Doubleday, 1995.

Kaiser, L. "Visionary Leadership." Speech given in workshop, "Visionary Leadership," during "Building Integrated Systems of Care," the 17th annual meeting of the Society for Healthcare Planning and Marketing of the American Hospital Association, Boston, Mass., May 8, 1995.

Kotter, J. P. *Leading Change*. Boston, Mass.: Harvard Business School Press, 1996.

Senge, P. M., and others. *The Fifth Discipline Fieldbook*. New York: Currency, 1994.

Whitley, E. M., and Heeley, G. F. "Integrity: More Than an Ounce of Prevention." *Spectrum*, Society for Healthcare Strategy and Market Development, July/Aug. 1998.

Chapter Three

Implementing Mission, Vision, and Values

Your mission, vision, and values drive your strategy, plans, and budgets. With the force and speed of change in today's society, it is more important than ever to define and implement a clear vision appropriately in order to achieve organizational goals, control costs, and deliver high-quality care. Four or five people at the senior management level cannot do it all. Dependence on your employees to fulfill the organization's mission requires that you provide them with clear goals so that they can do their jobs to the best of their ability. Nothing can be left to chance.

Writing the mission, vision, and values statements is the easy part. Getting from philosophy to strategy is more difficult. There are two activities involved: developing strategic goals and objectives and ensuring that individual actions are compatible with the stated mission, vision, and values.

Implementation does not happen naturally. You must work at defining each key word in the mission, vision, and values and the actions that represent them as an organization so that when key decisions need to be made, they can be made easily and quickly within the framework.

When every individual associated with the organization works in concert toward a common goal, the organization itself can become visionary, even without an individually charismatic leader. *Built to Last* (Collins and Porras, 1995) identified eighteen visionary companies that have achieved significant success over a long period without having a single identifiable visionary leader.

Visionary companies have been successful in very clearly defining the core ideology, goals, and objectives and the demanding standards expected of their employees. Then they go beyond this and do what others have not been so successful at—strictly holding each employee accountable for fulfilling the vision. While visionary companies are highly successful, they may not be the right place for everyone to work. Employees who perform their jobs and make decisions in accordance with the established vision will succeed and be rewarded. Employees who perform in contradiction to the established vision will be weeded out of the organization (Collins and Porras, 1995).

Health care organizations appear to be far behind other industries in their ability to clearly define goals and then act on them. This is due in part to the complexity of health care, which creates conflicted values, according to "Leadership for a Healthy 21st Century," a study conducted by the Health Forum, Arthur Andersen LLP, and DYG, Inc. "Healthcare is much more than the mere application of technology to diagnose and treat medical conditions. It is a complex business of relationships (among patients/consumers, family members, physicians/other providers, hospitals, employers/purchasers and payers) to optimize health, not just minimize illness. Healthcare, more than any other industry, lies at the 'intersection' of where we live, work and profit" (Mycek, 1998, pp. 26–30).

The study also found that health care leaders "say the right things about consumers and employees. In fact, they say the right things more than [others] do. But they don't act on them," according to Madelyn Hochstein, cofounder and president of DYG, Inc., which conducted the market research for the study (Mycek, 1998, pp. 26–30).

In this chapter, we will discuss developing and implementing appropriate strategic goals and objectives and how to ensure the compatibility of actions with mission, vision, and values.

Developing Strategy from Mission, Vision, and Values

In developing the organizational strategy from the philosophy of the mission, vision, and values, it is important to take the broad view and then become more specific as you move from strategy to goals, objectives, and action plans. The process needed to accomplish this, like developing the mission, vision, and values, is as unique as the organization but will include some broad "tried-and-true" techniques.

The first step is the development of the strategy. Mission, vision, and values drive the strategy (a careful plan or method), which then drives goals (the end toward which effort is directed), which drive objectives (the individual actions that together will achieve the goal), which are then used to create policies (definite courses or·methods of action to guide and determine present and future decisions selected from among alternatives in light of given conditions).

Once the strategy has been developed, implementation can begin. Implementation includes programs (the product lines and services provided), budgets (resources necessary to operate those programs), and procedures (how programs and policies are accomplished).

Most organizations end with implementation. However, it is important to review performance against previously set standards so that you can determine whether or not you have accomplished your goals. In this way, you will know whether your efforts have been effective in terms of both achieving goals and justifying the amount of time, energy, and other resources you invested.

To begin to move from mission, vision, and values to implementation, convene a strategic planning meeting of the organization's leadership group—senior management, board members, physicians, and others—to discuss the philosophy of your mission, vision, and values in the framework of workable strategies and an action plan. The group needs to discuss what steps are critical to realistically accomplish the vision. Annual leadership retreats, usually with outside facilitators, are common and effective techniques to accomplish this. Participants in a strategy development session should look at the factors outlined in Figure 3.1.

Figure 3.1. Questions for the Strategy Development Session.

- *Where are we now?* The situation: In all planning, participants must clearly understand at the outset the situation they confront because it is the launch pad for the future.

- *How did we get here?* The momentum: Given the situation, it is equally important to understand the nature of the forces that got the organization to its current status because these forces create momentum, and that momentum will carry the organization in a particular direction into the future.

- *Where are we going?* The momentum direction: Here the effort is one of projecting the organization into the future based on the nature and extent of the evident momentum.

- *Where should we be going?* The desired direction: Having articulated the apparent direction, planning participants assess its desirability. If necessary, a different and more attractive direction is determined.

- *How will we get there?* Strategy: Strategies and action plans are developed to accomplish the desired direction.

Source: Cinergy Services, Inc., 1998, p. 30.

Especially with a large group, an effective way to begin to combine a variety of opinions into a cohesive strategy is through the use of nominal group process, in which each person jots down goal ideas in four or five minutes. Ideas are then taken up one by one, one person at a time, and written on flip charts. Each idea is explained but no debate is permitted. Participants then vote on the action items using stick-on dots, which have different values. If you are concerned about certain participants unduly influencing others, you may choose to have participants vote independently on action items. When the votes are counted, the action items that receive the most support become the most important organizational goals and the items that receive the least support become secondary goals or are not chosen at all.

A key factor in developing strategies that will actually be able to be implemented is to keep them simple. Too often, health care organizations have multiple goals, some of which are in direct opposition to others. Beckham (1998, p. 60) affirms that an "effective strategic leader struggles with complexity and distills elegant simplicity. An irresistible vision. A single compelling strategic intent. A handful of clear strategies."

Beckham says that a strategic plan is concentrated.

> Too often, the strategic plan is burdened with a laundry list of initiatives. More than seven driving strategies usually suggests an unfocused mind. The result is "bunny planning," hopping off in thirteen directions without much effect. Tell a CEO an organization has too many strategies and you'll often get the same response, "You don't understand how complex our situation is." They are usually right about what the problem is—lack of understanding. If you can't get the number of strategies down to a handful, you haven't struggled enough with understanding your situation and your options.

Once the strategy and goals are defined, it is time to gain commitment for the strategic plan and allow middle managers and line employees to complete the formulation (objectives and policies) and design the implementation. Matejka (1991) outlines the "Seven C's" of the strategic commitment process shown in Figure 3.2.

Several other things are necessary, according to Matejka, to gain employee commitment, as outlined in Figure 3.3.

Once the strategic plan is developed and employee commitment is in place, it is the senior leadership's responsibility to "speak and act with consistency" according to Beckham (1998, p. 60). "Across time and place, a strategic leader demonstrates in words and actions that the strategic plan is alive in the organization. It is a ready point of reference for all important decisions. The question, 'How does this match up against our strategic plan?' is consistently asked by the CEO. The organization can see the strategic plan guiding critical decisions. The strategic leader becomes a manifest agent of the plan. Strategic leadership demands integrity. Integrity requires a CEO to speak and act with consistency."

Figure 3.2. Seven C's of the Strategic Commitment Process.

1. *Creating the Vision*. This is accomplished through the development of mission, vision, and values.

2. *Clarification*. The strategic plan clarifies mission, vision, and values.

3. *Connectedness*. The strategic plan defines the roles of individuals and groups within the organization and the interrelated tasks necessary to accomplish the plan.

4. *Communication*. The mission, vision, values, and strategic plan are carefully and consistently communicated to all employees within the organization so that they understand the importance of achievement and their individual role within the plan.

5. *Compensation*. There are individual and team rewards for accomplishment of the mission, vision, values, and strategic plan.

6. *Control*. Measurement and feedback mechanisms are in place to assess the progress that is made toward accomplishing the goals.

7. *Commitment*. Employees must believe that the organization's goal is their common goal. There has to be commitment from all levels of the organization that everyone pledge to carry out the common goal.

Source: Adapted from Matejka, 1991, pp. 184–186.

From Philosophy to Fulfillment

Consistent action is not just required of the CEO, but from everyone within the organization. Moving from the philosophy on paper to the fulfillment in action is a difficult thing for most of us to do. We deceive ourselves into believing that because we have defined our "lofty goals" in the mission, vision, and values statements that the little things will take care of themselves. However, as Kaiser (1995) has said, subtle dimensions of the organization may become the most important.

Visionary companies, as seen in *Built to Last* (Collins and Porras, 1995) use anecdotes and stories to create a corporate mythology. In fact, all companies have an anthology of stories that describe the culture of the organization. However, in many organizations, it is not quite so positive an influence.

What stories do your employees tell about your company? Are they positive or negative? Do they tell new employees, coworkers,

Figure 3.3. Additional Necessities to Gain Employee Commitment.

- *Respect.* There must be mutual respect between management and staff for their abilities to accomplish the goals. If either group lacks genuine respect for the other's ability to accomplish the goal, the plan is doomed to only partial accomplishment or complete failure.

- *Responsibility.* Each individual and group within the organization must accept responsibility for its portion of the plan's accomplishment. Individuals, groups, and senior management must also accept their responsibility to hold individuals and groups accountable for accomplishments. Some groups or individuals may have larger portions than others, but everyone is responsible for some portion of the plan and there must be accountability individually and as an organization.

- *Information.* The free flow of information is vital to accomplish strategic goals. Individuals and groups responsible for goal accomplishment need to have the information necessary to make decisions and take action. They also have the responsibility to ask for information that is not forthcoming.

- *Rewards.* Groups and individuals must be rewarded for goal accomplishment either through monetary reward or other type of recognition. A variety of recognition systems need to be in place because what works for one group or individual does not work for another. Likewise, negative consequences need to be in place for lack of accomplishment. This may be a lack of reward or more serious consequences, depending on the importance of the accomplishment.

- *Loyalty.* As with respect, loyalty must be cultivated within all levels of the organization. An organization's senior management cannot expect loyalty from its employees if it provides none first.

Source: Matejka, 1991, pp. 187–188.

family, and friends stories of heroism, values, and ethics? Or do they share stories of management incompetence and inconsistency, distrust, disloyalty, and lack of fair treatment? Would your organization's implementation of its mission, vision, and values through policies and procedures make a good "Dilbert" cartoon? Both positive and negative stories combine to form the mythology of the company and it begins at the senior levels of management.

Says Matejka (1991, p. 103), "Peter Drucker once said that the bottleneck is always at the head of the bottle. This statement has great meaning in organizations because . . . it is employees' perceptions regarding management that determine their behaviors. Fairness, consistency, and clarity in management actions and demands are critical to employee acceptance and performance."

How do you talk about employees and customers when they aren't around? Are you positive or negative? Do you publicly say that employees and customers are the hospital's most important assets and resources, but privately say that employees can't think for themselves or that customers are less than intelligent? Do you cultivate employees and promote from within for supervisory and management positions or hire from outside the organization? How do employees and customers fare in your budgets? Companies that truly put their money where their mouth is and respect, believe in, and trust their employees and customers are in turn treated with respect and trust.

Thoughts and words are powerful. What words do you use during difficult times or casual conversation? What words do you use in celebratory times? Are they sincerely felt and consistent with your mission, vision, and values? You create a self-fulfilling prophecy through your thoughts and expectations, which become words and actions. The best self-fulfilling prophecy is to treat people (patients, medical staff, employees, and the community) the way you expect them to act. How much time is spent worrying about and discussing past mistakes that cannot be changed rather than looking to the future and acting to create a different future?

You must turn values into daily practices—by living your values, by living your "words to live by." Again, it is not just the actions of senior leadership, but all employees throughout the organization. You can do this through consistency, constancy, and concentration.

As Kaiser (1995) has said, you create the future by your actions. What are the futures you are creating? What are the futures each individual employee is creating? You need to be creating the same—not conflicting—futures. This is why employee selection and rewarding positive behaviors are so important.

Too often, we do not do the difficult things because we want to be popular or well liked. A successful organization needs to develop collaborative traits among its employees, rather than individual, competitive concerns that only develop power struggles. You should reward behavior that is collaborative rather than competitive. Unfortunately, too often in health care power struggles are set up through allocation of budgets, FTEs, and departmental responsibilities. The organization is limited by the most restrictive thinking in it, which equals inaction or the wrong action as defined by its mission, vision, and values.

The Leadership Void

Too often, after senior leaders develop mission, vision, and values statements they continue to believe in them, regularly communicate them, but take for granted that managers, who are responsible for the actual implementation, are acting in accordance with the statements. They also sometimes underestimate the importance of the organization's reward systems that, more than anything else, will either enforce the mission, vision, and values or cause people to ignore the statements and act in ways that are inconsistent with stated goals.

Too often leaders who create a vision expect that the vision will be completed without the management of individual actions. Daily management of the vision is the next step—rewarding behaviors that achieve the vision and taking action when behaviors are contrary to the vision.

Many health care organizations embrace the values of trust, respect, honesty, and teamwork. However, there are many examples within those same organizations of rewards (or at least no negative consequences occurring) for behavior that is inconsistent with stated values. One example is when decisions made in a group meeting are changed as a result of the "meeting after the meeting." Some members of the group prefer to not work as a team or trust their coworkers by being honest in the work group, which in turn leads to a greater lack of trust. The rule should be: if it is not mentioned at the appropriate time and place, it receives no notice.

Another example of inconsistent actions is when an employee approaches a supervisor with a complaint about the actions of another employee, causing the supervisor to immediately become involved in the situation. Again, this shows a lack of trust that conflicts cannot be resolved in an adult, civilized manner between the two individuals involved. The supervisor's first question in this situation needs to be, "And what did she say when you brought this to her attention?" Confronting situations head on, while initially painful, will only result in more positive outcomes in the long run.

One CEO new to a small, rural hospital began implementing changes he felt necessary to turn the hospital's image and financial position around. He enjoyed a number of successes, but also some resistance to his efforts. In discussing necessary changes with the department head of a clinical area, the department head said she would be uncomfortable and unable to implement the CEO's changes. He suggested that in that case, this hospital was probably not an appropriate place for her to continue to work. The department head agreed and gave her notice.

The next day, having thought about her decision, she went back to the CEO and asked to withdraw her resignation. The CEO asked her if she would now be able to agree to and implement the necessary changes in the department. When she declined, he replied that her resignation was still effective. He said, "If I had caved in and let her stay, it would have sent the wrong message to the rest of the employees who were implementing the necessary changes."

At McMurry Publishing in Phoenix, one of the company values is, "Deliver raving customer service." Several years ago, in order to keep a customer happy, an employee offered 20,000 free magazines. Says CEO Preston McMurry, "So, the question arises, was that the right thing to do? Or would we have been better off trying to pacify the customer with 5,000 free magazines? To my mind the question is moot, for the customer was very happy. And since delivering raving customer service is one of our values, I couldn't have been more pleased with the result" (*Inside McMurry*, 1998). (For more about McMurry Publishing's implementation of corporate values, see the case study that concludes this chapter.)

Matejka (1991, p. 157) makes this point:

> Management and leadership are slightly different, mostly related, and certainly needed in combination. A leader is someone who takes initiative, and a manager is someone who guides. Hardly a huge difference. In fact, it would seem that both capacities are necessary if one is to be an effective person. Initiating action without the skill to guide the accomplishment is foolhardy. Likewise, guiding activities without the vision to initiate can sometimes be counterproductive. Certainly leaders need vision to initiate action. We need more leaders. A leader can, however, be a fighter or healer, a builder or a destroyer. And a manager who "guides" expertly would seem to be initiating action toward a vision. To some people, leadership sounds more exciting. But remember, the true difference lies in the proven "vision" of effective leaders.

The myth of visionary leaders, as pointed out in *Built to Last*, is that a successful company requires a charismatic leader. In fact, the authors found that the opposite was the case. Most highly successful organizations rarely had the traditional charismatic leader, but had developed a culture of vision that was so strong that it survived long after the departure of the founder and even after multiple top executives (Collins and Porras, 1995, p. 23).

What happens when an individual in the senior management ranks disagrees with the stated mission, vision, and values, is self-motivated, and is organizationally destructive? What penalties exist in the organization to prevent this behavior?

Too often, we punish people who do the right thing. We may say we want intelligent patients who will be involved in their treatment, yet we consider patients who want information "difficult."

We may say we seek change agents, but being a change agent in many organizations is not a good long-term employment situation. In fact, it may be a career-shortening decision, as expressed by Himmelman (1998, p. 41): "Being identified as a person willing to challenge existing institutional cultures, practices and power relations is not the best strategy for upward mobility in most organizations."

Whatever your organization's mission, vision, and values, it can begin to create its preferred culture by

- Recognizing the fulfillment of mission, vision, and values as a leadership issue. The presence of a passive leader who has high personal standards is not sufficient. The leader's responsibility is to define, promote, and perpetuate the mission, vision, and values of the organization.

- Being explicit about your mission, values, and commitments. The identity of your organization should make sense and be taken seriously.

- Defining, evaluating, and rewarding success. And individuals who exemplify the mission, vision, and values should be recognized.

- Constructing the necessary structures and providing resources that support mission, vision, and values.

- Evaluating prospective employees for endorsement of their ability to fulfill the mission, vision, and values.

- Implementing education and training programs for all employees and investing in leadership development to fulfill mission, vision, and values (adapted from Whitley and Heeley, 1998, pp. 4–5).

If you need to develop trust within your organization, you may want to consider the Behavioral Trust and Change Program (Figure 3.4) developed by Ken Matejka (1991).

Figure 3.4. Behavioral Trust and Change Program.

- *Judge the fit.* If you feel such a program is valuable to your organization, adapt these steps to fit your own organization's individual needs.

- *Build a success story.* Start small so that employees can see results. You will build trust gradually, but small successes count and should be celebrated.

- *Choose the behavior you want.* Identify only specific, observable, performance-related behavior. Do not judge behavior according to your own biases, but on mutually agreed on values that will lead the organization to its goals.

- *Monitor when, where, and how often the behavior occurs.* Some behavior occurs as a result of external factors. Any time a consistent pattern occurs, the behavior is not capricious. Find out what the reasons for the behavior are.

- *Consider the present consequences of the behavior.* Most people act in rational ways to maximize pleasure and minimize pain. Maybe the consequence isn't important to the employee. Perhaps the consequence is actually encouraging the behavior. Often, we reward disruptive employees with transfers to more desirable assignments just to get rid of them. Sometimes we give employees our attention when they misbehave. Analyze the situation. What is the employee's motivation?

- *Hold exchange meetings with your people.* Share information, expectations, perceptions, and goals and find reasonable, workable solutions that are mutually beneficial. Talk about the mission, vision, and values frequently throughout the organization, both formally and informally. Create a book club with supervisory and management staff meeting regularly to read and discuss the organizational implications of a book on leadership, management, or some other issue.

- *Choose and communicate your strategies.* Formulate and establish the best strategies for behavioral change. Make sure that both rewards and punishments for behavior have the desired effect.

- *Check the resulting behavior.* Monitor, measure, and record whatever the performance indicators are. Having employees measure their own performance makes them more aware of their performance and how it affects others and the achievement of organizational goals.

- *Deliver what you promised.* This is the most important aspect of building trust—by showing the employee and any interested observers what happens when someone performs well or poorly.

- *Regroup.* Evaluate results against desired performance and changes in the environment. Make necessary adjustments and revisions.

Source: Adapted from Matejka, 1991, pp. 104–106.

Doing Well for Yourself by Doing Good
for the Organization

Although the author of the following statement is unknown, it is still applicable to the achievement of organizational goals: "There is no limit to the good a man can do if he doesn't care who gets the credit." Too often, individuals within organizations act in their own personal interest, rather than in the interests of the organization that pays their salary.

As Fellers (1994, p. 10) says,

> Things go wrong in business because we make many decisions with fear, politics, lack of knowledge and personal agendas lurking just beneath the surface. These problems are like cutoff tree trunks in a lake. The stumps are under the water ready to wreck the boat at any moment. The water level rises and falls uncontrollably as a result of economic conditions and uncertainty within the firm. Instead of eliminating the stumps, we often just try raising the water level a little to buy some time. As a result, the larger good of both the firm and its employees often suffer when we eliminate symptoms—not the causes behind why things go wrong.

Things also go wrong because managers and leaders at times lack the strength of leadership. In her book *Jesus, CEO* Jones (1995) outlines three categories of leadership strength. Success in management and leadership requires the total combination:

- *Strength of self-mastery.* "If you have not been tested by fire, you do not know who you are. And if you do not know who you are, you cannot be a leader" (p. 5).
- *Strength of action.* Everything and everyone is alive and full of possibilities. "Leaders should have more confidence, because everything is alive!" (p. 82).
- *Strength of relationships.* "History repeatedly has shown that people hunger for something larger than themselves. Leaders

who offer that will have no shortage of followers. In fact, higher purpose is such a vital ingredient to the human psyche that as Scripture says, 'Where there is no vision, the people perish.' Studies show that people will work harder and longer on projects when they understand the overall significance of their individual contribution" (pp. 177–178).

The following are three different kinds of leadership styles commonly used in companies, including health care institutions:

- *Authoritarianism.* Employees are told (rather than asked) to "do it" without sufficient information about the goals, objectives, and reasoning behind the action. Without sufficient information and understanding, employees may accomplish the task, but in a manner opposed to the manager's intent. This causes not only rework, but lack of trust and hard feelings on everyone's part.
- *Micromanagement.* On the opposite end of the spectrum, employees are told (again, rather than asked) exactly how to do something. This also undermines trust, leading employees to think that the manager does not believe they have the sufficient skills or intelligence to complete the task.
- *Collaboration.* In this leadership style, managers and employees work together to accomplish the task. Management provides sufficient information about the goals and the broad parameters for what is to be accomplished, and employees can use their knowledge, skills, and experience to accomplish it.

The complexity of issues affecting health care today are such that neither an authoritarian decree nor micromanagement will serve the organization well because too much effort is required on the part of a few individuals in management positions.

To get the beneficial effects of a visionary organization like the ones profiled in *Built to Last* (Collins and Porras, 1995), you must build your organization into one that preserves your philosophy in specific ways. The following send a consistent set of reinforcing signals that indoctrinate people and create a sense of belonging:

- Training programs that have an ideological as well as a practical slant
- On-the-job socializing
- Promoting from within
- Penalties for acting in ways contradictory to the mission, vision, and values
- Constant emphasis on corporate values and heritage and tales of heroic deeds in the line of duty

Such methods pay. Visionary companies create cult-like cultures built around an ideology of turning people loose knowing they'll do things that will achieve organizational goals within its mission, vision, and values.

Operational managers who rarely have input into the development of mission, vision, and values statements or the development of the actual strategic plan can develop departmental strategies from these corporate statements through an easy six-step process. Operational managers, including those responsible for human resources and marketing, should ask themselves these questions about the organization:

1. *What* do you do?
2. *Who* do you do it for?
3. *How* do you do it better than others?
4. *When* do customers need your products and services?
5. *Where* do customers obtain your products or services?
6. *Why* do customers need your product; why should they buy your products or services rather than your competitors'?

From these questions, managers can create individual departmental action plans that fit within the framework of the mission, vision, and values. From a marketing perspective, knowing who your customers are, when they need your service, and where they obtain it will help you develop marketing strategies that fit the customer's needs and are written in the customer's language. From a human resources perspective, knowing what you do and who you do it for will help you identify the right employees to provide your customers with the service they desire.

The traditional placement of human resources and marketing as separate functions has worked for health care (and other) organizations in the past. However, with a rapidly changing economy and work environment, more of the organization's success is dependent on a workforce that must think quickly and independently—an information-based workforce. Integrating marketing and human resources functions within an organization will allow both functions to work more efficiently and effectively to achieve organizational goals. The next chapter will look at the forces driving this integration.

Case Study:
Living the Mission at McMurry Publishing, Inc.

McMurry Publishing, Inc.,* has implemented several practices that serve to keep the company's mission and values in front of employees and reward them for living the company philosophy. CEO Preston McMurry is a firm believer in the philosophy that "your employees won't treat your clients any better than you treat them." And it permeates throughout the company—in the mission and

---

*This case study is based on interviews with Christopher M. McMurry, chief operating officer, McMurry Publishing, Inc., Phoenix, Arizona, October 1998; and Preston McMurry, chief executive officer, December 1998. The information on open-book management and profit sharing is based on the fall 1998 issue of *Inside McMurry*.

values communicated to all employees in a variety of ways, Monday morning meetings, an integrated evaluation process, open-book management, and a five-step interview process to make sure the right people are hired. Established as an independent business in 1989, McMurry publishes high-quality custom and syndicated magazines and has achieved tremendous growth since Preston purchased the company from the hospital corporation that founded it in 1984—from two employees in 1989 to seventy-five in 1998 and from revenue of less than $500,000 in 1989 to $17 million in 1998. Its health care titles include *Vim & Vigor*, *eHealth*, *Health Direct*, and *Smart Health*.

Mission and Values

McMurry's mission and values are communicated to each new employee in a variety of ways, including the employee handbook. New employees are asked to sign a copy of the company's eight values and each receives an orientation to the McMurry value system in a three-hour discussion and exchange of ideas. The values discussion continues each week at the mandatory Monday morning meeting.

Monday Morning Meetings

Each Monday, the work week begins with a one-hour meeting that serves as both training and communication session. McMurry invests a significant amount of staff time and money into these meetings, which range from training programs by outside speakers to general company announcements or reports by departments about what they do and how they do it. Regardless of what is on the agenda, there is always a discussion about the mission and values.

"Values should be simple so that people can remember what they are, but they can also be very vague," says COO Christopher (Chris) McMurry. "So we have these sessions on Monday morning and talk about how people interpret 'Do the right thing' or other values. They express what they think it means, but they also learn how other people interpret that value." This process creates common definitions for the McMurry values, which in turn "create an environment in which everyone understands how they should behave—a code of conduct. You can't create a code without specific identifiable values. By having a broader discussion about a particular value, people become more enlightened and it narrows the definition and enhances the understanding."

Says Preston, "Without fail, we address the issue of customer service. Everyone is required to come to the meeting with some customer service experience from the past week and be prepared to relate it to McMurry Publishing and our value system. It's the constant drip that wears the rock thin."

Independent Decision Making

As a result of this consistent discussion of mission and values, employees are capable of making decisions without constantly seeking management approval. Says Preston,

> I don't want employees asking me what to do. I don't even want employees to come to me with solutions. I want employees who come to me and say "This is what I did." I want employees who make their own decisions. I had an employee come to me very early on and ask which of two beautiful pictures I preferred for the cover of *Vim & Vigor*. I knew which one I preferred and I love choosing the best picture. But I won't do that. It's their job and I want them to make their own decisions. Because if I make their decisions, number one, they will never learn and number two, they will do it for me rather than themselves. You make the best decisions when you work for yourself.

McMurry's employee handbook states, "It's vitally important to understand these values because they are fundamental to performance evaluations. In addition, it's expected that each staff member will base decisions, actions and behaviors upon McMurry's eight-point value system. Remember, and this is important, there has never been an occasion in which a staff member has been admonished for an error, when a judgment was based upon one or more of McMurry's values."

There are many examples of this at McMurry and the stories are told among employees as part of the organization's folklore. Preston firmly believes, "You've never met anyone in your life who says, 'I can't wait to go to work and screw up.' When you think about the decisions people make during the course of a day, they make very few mistakes. But every once in a while, someone makes a mistake. And when they make a mistake, it's a matter of opinion or degree. There are usually many dozens of correct answers and many of those will work as well as others. The decisions that an employee makes will generally not bankrupt the company."

And what about when it could bankrupt the company? Preston even has a story about a big financial mistake that was made. The decision to "do the right thing" resulted in sticking with the employee, who has since become an extremely valuable team member.

Evaluation System

Another step in the process to incorporate the organization's mission and values into the daily lives of employees is the McMurry evaluation process. The evaluation tool used is the eight-point value statement and employees are asked to write out the mission statement. There are no boxes to check; the evaluator is simply required to think about how the values are being lived.

"I just completed one evaluation that was twelve pages long," said Chris. "For instance, on the value 'produce quality always' I wanted to get across to the employee that an element of quality is preparation—not just creating a fancy, nice-looking product."

Chris says it is not possible "to get people to live out the values if they're not measured against them. By connecting the values to how people are evaluated, it forces people to pay attention to them, to learn what they really mean, to live them out, and make their decisions day-to-day based on those values. We've all worked for companies where the mission was hung on a wall and no one paid much attention to it once it was crafted and made into a plaque. This is a way to take it off the wall and put it at the top of people's minds."

Open-Book Management and Profit Sharing

The final facet of McMurry's tenacious implementation of mission and values is open-book management (OBM), which is intrinsically related to the firm's value system and its long-range plan. The value system, for example, calls for staff members to "do the right thing" and to "deliver raving customer service always." More specifically, the OBM program is designed to benefit customers first and then reward staff members for making their day. It is a can't-miss strategy that saves customers money and shares profits with a staff motivated to retain customers and grow the business by attracting new ones.

The combination of treating both customers and staff well produces remarkable results, including increased profits. It's a win-win plan.

Six departments are set up as virtual businesses; that is to say, they have their own set of books, profit and loss, and bottom line. Virtual business managers run their own show, make their own decisions including when to hire, what to pay, how to address problems, and how much to spend on marketing. They share the cost of central services. All they have to do is make the bottom line and maintain the McMurry value system.

Each quarter, all staff members receive complete financials for their department, including a profit and loss statement. Then, following a week-long opportunity to study their financials, each department's staff members meet to discuss the quarter's results with their department manager and prepare for their meeting with McMurry's CFO, COO, and president. It is here that each staff member is required to come prepared to ask at least one financial question and discuss costs, revenues, problems, growth, and cost-saving opportunities. And last but not least, quarterly bonus checks are handed out, each individual department member sharing equally in his or her department's bottom line.

OBM delivers the goods for McMurry. It works because top management takes an ongoing, active interest in making it happen, motivating staff top to bottom, and insisting that everyone get involved in a very real way. McMurry staffers average an additional 16 percent compensation from the bonus program.

A teamwork survey, done two years in a row, shows improvements in departmental operations and the ability of individual departments to work together. Also, after the distribution of the *Staff Handbook* in mid-1998, a test to analyze employees' comprehension of the handbook material uncovered an interesting correlation. The highest scores correlated to the most well-run departments.

The results for McMurry have been extraordinary. Turnover is low—in fact, over the past year, several McMurry staff members who left to explore other opportunities have returned to the company. Success over the past twelve years can be measured not only in company growth by the traditional revenue measurement, but also in the rising number of employees, magazine titles, and applicants for open positions. Growth would not have been this great without the full integration of mission and values.

"We've had people apply for jobs here three or five times before they may get hired. Two of our publications are a direct result of people who didn't get hired here, but who came back with ideas for magazines for their new employers," says Preston.

References

Beckham, D. "The Hunger for Strategic Leadership." *Healthcare Forum Journal*, Sept./Oct. 1998.

Cinergy Services, Inc. *Building Healthy Communities*. Plainfield, Ind.: Cinergy Corporation, 1998.

Collins, J. C., and Porras, J. I. *Built to Last: Successful Habits of Visionary Compa-nies*. New York: HarperCollins, 1995.

Fellers, G. *Why Things Go Wrong: Deming Philosophy in a Dozen Ten-Minute Ses-sions*. New York: Pelican Books, 1994.

Himmelman, A. "Inside/Out: Change Agents and Community Partnerships." *Healthcare Forum Journal*, July/Aug. 1998.

Inside McMurry, spring 1998.

Jones, L. B. *Jesus, CEO*. New York: Hyperion, 1995.

Kaiser, L. "Visionary Leadership." Speech given in workshop, "Visionary Lead-ership," during "Building Integrated Systems of Care," the 17th annual meeting of the Society for Healthcare Planning and Marketing of the American Hospital Association, Boston, Mass., May 8, 1995.

Matejka, K. *Why This Horse Won't Drink: How to Win—and Keep—Employee Commitment*. New York: AMACOM, 1991.

Mycek, S. "Leadership for a Healthy 21st Century." *Healthcare Forum Journal*, July/Aug. 1998.

Whitley, E. M., and Heeley, G. F. "Integrity: More Than an Ounce of Preven-tion." *Spectrum*, Society for Healthcare Strategy and Market Develop-ment, July/Aug. 1998.

Chapter Four

Linking Human Resources
and Marketing

Health care is more than technology, tests, and drugs. Health care is human, individual, and personal in a way that technology can never be. The actual provision of health care is the art in the "art and science" of medicine. The human touch of health care is one of the few things your patients and families truly understand about their health care experience. It is the best way your customers know how to judge the quality of the care they receive.

For a nurse, taking care of the family of a dying cancer patient can become as important as maintaining the patient's comfort—explaining the unexplainable disease process, offering a hug in comfort, sharing her personal experience with death and dying. For a doctor, taking a few extra minutes to make sure that the patient and family understand the purpose of a test, what to expect, and what the possible outcomes are can make a huge difference in the patient's anxiety level as well as his or her compliance with tests and treatments. Remembering that you are not just treating a disease but caring for a person ensures that the patient understands that you care.

Employees who provide direct patient care understand this because they experience it every day. But it is easy for those who work in offices and spend their days in meetings to forget their fundamental mission.

Every business is dependent on its employees' performance to make and deliver the product and interact with customers. In a service industry like health care the employee's behavior is the product. Hiring, training, and retaining the type of employees who will help you achieve your organizational goals will move you closer to the customer than large marketing expenditures will. However, in health care it often appears that considerably more money is spent on marketing (advertising, sales, and public relations) than on the employees who truly shape your public image.

Out with the Old

The role of both marketing and human resources departments has changed with the shifting views about personnel and the organization, the changing role of government, new electronic networks, and the enormous changes in society in general. Professionals who want to survive and thrive need to align their personal career goals with the business goals of the organization.

With increasing competition and customer expectations, shorter technical innovation and product life cycles, and other forces changing the rules for success, it is becoming increasingly clear that the best hope for sustainable competitive advantage is in people. It is imperative for human resources and marketing functions to break old patterns, go beyond their traditional supporting roles, and increase their credibility as contributors to strategic business solutions. The key to future success will be to consistently add value to the product by becoming a business partner with other departments and consult with each of them and the line managers to align strategies, processes, and practices with business needs.

As stated in Chapter 1, the terms *marketing* and *human resources* are defined more broadly in this book than they would be by most health care administrators. Traditionally, health care marketing departments have been responsible for creating and maintaining the organization's image through advertising, public relations, customer service programs, and other promotional activities. True marketing involves both the internal systems, which affect the delivery of service to consumers, and the traditional external activities, which result in leads and referrals to the organization—writing, design, layout, desktop publishing, advertising, and market research.

The term *human resources* has also suffered from a narrow definition in health care: that of primarily being the administration of policies and procedures, compensation, benefits, safety reporting, legal requirements, and other operational and bureaucratic tasks. In reality, human resources professionals are best used in an organization in a strategic function to design formal systems that ensure the effective and efficient use of human talent to accomplish organizational goals. Human resources professionals have significant experience in the areas of employee relations, training and development, and employee selection. They are able to assess the internal environment and understand the expectations of current and prospective employees.

The traditional "silo" organizational chart also isolates what the functions of these departments can do. Neither marketing nor human resource management is an isolated function, but a set of activities that must be accomplished throughout the organization, not just by the individuals within a particular department. Marketing—identifying the customer's needs and then satisfying them—should be a daily part of each employee's job. Human resource management—ensuring the effective and efficient use of human capital to accomplish organizational goals—should be the responsibility of each manager and each employee throughout the organization.

The Current View

In 1996 the American Hospital Association (AHA) conducted an extensive research project called "Reality $\sqrt{}$" (American Hospital Association, 1996), which used focus groups and opinion research to study the public's perception of health care and the role hospitals play in health care delivery.

The results were, if not shocking, at least disturbing to those who still believe that the basic mission of hospitals is to treat the ill, comfort the dying, and prevent illness whenever possible. The Executive Summary of the study reported, "The public is deeply concerned and troubled about changes occurring in health care and hospitals. They feel a growing impact upon themselves and their families in terms of reduced access, higher costs, lower quality, the competence of care givers and a trend toward impersonal care. They see a growing focus on the financial 'bottom line' overwhelming what they believe should be a dedication to individual patient care."

In 1997, the AHA followed up with "Reality √ II" (American Hospital Association, 1997–1998), which reported the following results:

- The public's perception of why organizational changes occur is hospital profit. Patients see little benefit from mergers and acquisitions to them, the care they receive, or the community.

- The patient's definition of quality is the nurse (broadly defined by the public as any of a number of caregivers, including RNs, LPNs, nursing assistants, or even respiratory therapists or nutritionists). Patients recognize that there are fewer bedside nurses, and the ones who are on the units are overworked and hampered by hospital bureaucracy and insurers. However, some patients are reluctant to be referred to a physician assistant or nurse practitioner rather than a physician for their first medical contact.

- The increasing corporatization of health care structure, behavior, language, and communication strongly conflicts with people's deep-seated perception of health care as a human service that touches their hopes, fears, and deepest emotions.

- Increasingly, patients view no one as their advocate in an industry that is riddled with waste, fraud, and abuse.

- Patients' perceptions of hospitals are the products of their personal experiences, not the products of a marketing department's creative process. There is significant skepticism or outright disbelief about most hospital advertising, unless the aim is to convey health information and availability of services. Image advertising was most often dismissed and regarded as a factor in increasing health care costs. And advertising is another example of hospitals and health systems mistakenly presenting their messages to consumers using business terms instead of quality-of-care terms.

- The public also can easily separate institutions from people. The people who work in hospitals always are viewed as good, caring people while the institution that surrounds them may or may not be viewed as positively.

There are two common reactions to such negative news about our industry. The first is a form of denial in which we rationalize the information within the context of our organization and explain away the objections: "That's not us. Those focus groups were probably done in (some state far away)." "If people really knew us, they wouldn't say that about us. But it's true about our competition." "People just don't realize how complex health care is. It's just not as easy as other industries."

The second common reaction asks a department functioning in isolation from other departments to fix the problem. For instance, after receiving the "Reality √" report, a senior executive of one health care organization asked the hospital marketing director, "What are you planning on doing to combat that perception?"

In with the New

Neither denial nor simple delegation will resolve the public's lack of trust in health care organizations. Only the deliberate actions of committed and caring employees, along with the support of senior leadership, will regain the lost trust. The AHA is continuing its "Reality √" project to provide information to member hospitals about the public's perceptions of the industry. With the current health care climate, one department cannot be the sole caretaker of the organization's image. The multiple forces bearing down on health care require an integrated effort among all departments, with marketing and human resources departments leading the way to take advantage of the similarities in their functions as well as capitalize on their unique abilities in a synergistic approach.

Intellectual Capital

According to Steve Wallam, president of the Securities and Exchange Commission, "In 10 years, measures of intellectual capital will become the most closely watched numbers in annual reports" (Russell, 1999, p. 50).

The traditional measurements of corporate value—assets and liabilities, revenue and expenses, profit margin, ratio, and return on investment—are still important, but they are no longer the only meaningful measures of performance for companies in an information and technology age. Training, customer and employee retention and satisfaction, quality, new product development, and other factors are becoming more and more important to companies in a variety of industries.

In an information society, a business must measure its worth better "by checking not only last quarter's profits, but also counting the brains it can bring to bear on the process in the current quarter: its so-called intellectual capital, its training, its employee retention—in short, its people and their capabilities, and how well they mesh" (Hequet, 1996, p. 42).

According to *Management Review*, all eight crucial factors for success in the information age are intangible. "Companies must generate passion, constantly reinvent themselves, build focus and concentration, devote themselves to service excellence, adapt to change, respond quickly, be flexible and build trust" (Hequet, 1996, p. 45).

Changing focus is necessary for health care institutions to regain the trust of their customers and communities. As we have said before, investment in customer satisfaction and employee retention is essential to their success. We repeat this again because it is too important to forget. It is time to adequately and appropriately measure and invest in these two vital factors in our success.

"Leadership for a Healthy 21st Century," a study undertaken by Health Forum, Arthur Andersen, and DYG (1999), recommends a new model for health care accounting that takes into consideration physical assets, financial assets, customer assets, and provider (employee) assets. Recommendations for how to measure the intangible customer and provider assets are also included (p. 7). This report encourages health care organizations "to begin their own initiatives to develop information into what creates value, and how these tangible and intangible assets can be invested in and managed to benefit all stakeholders" (p. 13).

Shifting focus from money to people will be difficult for some in the health care arena. According to Hequet (1996, p. 47), "top brass has clutched at currency so long they may have forgotten that people do the work."

It will probably be difficult for senior managers who were traditionally trained in the financial aspects of health care administration to shift their thinking to the new intangible measurements of success. This is where the marketing and human resources professionals enter the picture. The HR and marketing departments are familiar with dealing with intangibles—how employee morale improves when a new benefit is introduced or how much goodwill is created by a community health program. Teaching financially based administrators how to measure intangibles will be a key task for HR and marketing professionals.

Human Resources and Marketing: Similarities

The ability to measure and define how intangibles create value for an organization is only the beginning of the similarities among human resources and marketing professionals. Others include supporting the organization's mission, a dedication to customer service excellence, organizational and market alignment, and an ability to deal with customers with a variety of experience and knowledge. In addition, both disciplines speak as the conscience of the organization, representing employees and the public when organizational policies and special interests are contradictory.

First and most important, both functions support the mission and operational goals of the organization. Without employees (human resources), the delivery of care could not occur, nor would there be any differentiation from competition. Without a continuing base of customer support and nurturing of new customers (marketing), the organization could not maintain or grow its business.

Customer Service Excellence

There are many examples across the country of excellent partnerships between training and organizational development staff actively working with marketing and public relations staff in implementing a customer service program. The marketing staff are aware of customer expectations globally and within individual markets and—from patient satisfaction surveys—what their own patients expect. Training staff can assist in the planning and implementation of employee development activities, whether setting up specific customer service training programs or incorporating the topic within other training programs that meet organizational goals.

Both human resources and marketing department staff must have a strategic commitment to transforming the hospital's culture by institutionalizing and sustaining an environment of customer service excellence. Not only do the departments' staff need to help define customer service standards and teach them to others, they need to model the behavior themselves daily.

Too often employees are hired for clinical competence and it is assumed that the employee has the requisite customer service skills to perform his or her job. This is a dangerous assumption to make because each individual defines good customer service in a different way. The golden rule doesn't really apply in service delivery. "Do unto others as you would have them do unto you" leaves too much room for misinterpretation.

An employee who prefers to be treated formally when in the "customer" role may call a patient "Mr." or "Mrs." Another employee who prefers to be more informal may call the patient by his or her first name. Each one is making an assumption about the patient's preference.

It is very important to remember one of the corollaries to customer service: customer service is how most patients define quality. Patients expect a minimum quality standard; they expect that every professional in the organization has the clinical skills to do his or her job. In fact, quality is simply the price of admission to get into the show; it is a given. What will begin to differentiate one health care organization from another is service. Most people cannot evaluate the technical competence of staff. Instead they rely on such intangible factors as how professional the caregivers appear, their behavior, and the way they treat the patient and family from a service perspective (respect, privacy, dignity).

Marketing can assist in identifying the behavior expected by the consumer, and training and development staff can provide the education content. A combination of employees can present the actual training. Human resources staff can identify and develop strategies to link customer service behavior with ongoing performance standards and the organization's performance appraisal system. Finally, marketing and training together can develop the external standards of measurement to determine whether the training was effective.

Alignment

Alignment may be defined as the proper positioning or state of adjustment of parts. Marketing and human resources professionals deal with the issue of alignment on a daily basis. The role of marketing is to gather information about customer needs and align those needs with the strengths of the organization to develop products and services needed by the marketplace. Marketing is responsible for helping the organization understand the alignment between its preferred image and its actual image in the community. Human resource systems ensure alignment by focusing on the organization's needs to provide services and the appropriate employees to meet those needs. They also seek to align employee needs for competitive wages and benefits with the organization's financial stability.

An area of alignment between the two functions that has been sorely underutilized is between customer needs and hiring the appropriate employees to perform those functions. Traditionally the focus of employee recruitment has been on the clinical aspects of the job, which, of course, are quite important. But from a customer standpoint, clinical competence is a given; customers expect more. Your goal should be to become an organization focused on customer needs and staffed by employees who understand not only the clinical aspects of their jobs but also customer needs, the organization's goals, how to meet customer needs, and how to accomplish organizational goals.

The key to building alignment, according to Cobb, Samuel, and Sexton (1998, p. 34), is "changing organization and employee behaviors (the province of HR) in coordination with an in-depth understanding of change in a dynamic global marketplace (the province of marketing)."

Customer Focus

Both marketing and human resources professionals are customer focused; they recognize both internal and external customers and their needs. Some marketing departments may be too heavily focused on external markets and pay too little attention to internal marketing and communications (a subject we will discuss in detail in Chapter 9). Likewise, some human resources departments may be too heavily focused on a certain segment of their internal customers (who are interested in finance and holding down costs) rather than on the needs of the employee group as a whole (employee morale and retention). A balance between internal and external customers must be reached within both functions.

We have heard the term *internal and external customers* so often that sometimes we forget what it truly means. We define the concept to mean that every employee within an organization should focus his or her efforts on helping those employees who are meeting the needs of external customers—our patients and their families.

It is easy for hospital administrators and other employees to get caught up in the mundane tasks of their jobs and believe that their efforts are important, when in fact they may have little impact on the actual external customer. Not only do the minutiae of regulations, managed care, and financial pressures often distract us from our true mission, they may also completely overshadow it. Let's be honest. How does writing a quality report or sitting in yet another meeting looking at financial or human resource data help the patient in room 302B?

If what you are doing is not directly meeting the needs of an external customer or making it easier or more pleasant for another person within the organization to meet the needs of an external customer: *Stop doing it!*

Internal Communication

Internal communication is probably one of the more common interactions between marketing and human resources departments. The purpose of internal communication has traditionally been to provide information to employees on activities, events, benefits, and other employment issues through a printed newsletter. However, internal communication is also incredibly valuable in communicating organizational goals and accomplishments and should include marketing activities. These communication pieces are not often used to truly give employees the tools they need to serve as ambassadors for the organization.

The human resources department is the source of many, if not most, employee communications, whereas the marketing department has the expertise in communications media and theory to determine the best method of dissemination.

As we will discuss in Chapter 9, employee communication does not have to be limited to printed materials. In fact, ad hoc focus groups or continuing employee relations councils can provide a feedback loop to validate the effectiveness of communication as well as process implementation. This type of group communication, especially when coordinated between HR and marketing, has a significant effect on the organizational culture. Employees are able to communicate how the implementation is progressing or how the communication of a process is being received directly to the persons who designed the process.

Working with Other Departments

Both departments are already working with the same people in their support of other departments throughout the organization. Marketing assists clinical departments in marketing services, helps all departments with customer service and image issues, and provides feedback from patient satisfaction surveys. HR staff works with these same departments to hire and train employees, handle employee relations issues, and administer compensation and benefits programs.

There could also be some overlap in functional responsibilities. In some organizations, the volunteer services department may report to the marketing area because it is seen as a valuable community relationship or fund-raising group that should be nurtured. In other organizations, volunteers are seen as human resources, equal in value to employees, and thus report to the HR department. Regardless of which department has responsibility for this function, they should be working together to use volunteers effectively throughout the organization and the community.

Similar Tools

A final similarity is that both functions use similar methods in approaching problems, finding solutions, and gathering information. Environmental assessments, customer needs analysis, focus groups, surveys, interviews, communicating with multiple publics, and, finally, planning, organizing, and evaluating strategies and projects are common to professionals in both functions.

Human Resources and Marketing: Differences

Despite the similarities in goals and functions, there are some significant differences between the two areas. Language and perceptions are two that come immediately to mind.

Each profession has its own language. HR professionals frequently talk in acronyms (FSLA, ADA, FMLA) and bureaucratic terms (performance appraisal, grievance procedure, exit interview). Marketing professionals speak in terms of quantitative research, market share, ad space, direct mail, and collateral materials. This is not to say that it is not possible or even likely to be able to bridge the language gap—in fact it is done every day.

Human resources professionals are often perceived as bureaucratic paper administrators and managers, focused on internal customers. Marketing professionals are often perceived as either temperamental creative types or narrowly focused data crunchers too focused on the external audience.

Negative Similarities

Given the vast similarities between human resources and marketing and the few differences, what are the reasons these two functions have rarely before gotten together to achieve organizational goals? It has to do with negative similarities, which are not necessarily unique to these functions but, unfortunately, are widespread throughout hospital organizations.

The first negative similarity is the lack of understanding of what the other department does, coupled with a lack of willingness to learn. As one group of authors investigating the linkage between the two said, "(they) are not only not integrated but in fact rarely talk to each other. They might even claim to not understand each other" (Cobb, Samuel, and Sexton, 1998, p. 32). In some organizations, this can be directly related to a lack of trust between departments (the "*we* work harder than any other department around here, and I have no idea what *they* do all day" syndrome).

This lack of understanding is closely related to turf protection. Some mid-level managers and even some senior level executives reason: if you don't know what I do (and vice versa) then you can't take over. However, this turf protection—allowed to permeate hospitals through departmental isolation—causes duplication of effort and barriers to achieving full personal, professional, and organizational potential. Of course, the internal systems within the organization must be in place to reward working together rather than protecting turf. A health care organization that rewards department managers according to the size of their budget, number of FTEs, and other traditional measurement tools is generally not an organization that rewards departmental collaboration.

This question begs the greater question of whether or not you understand the rewards that you bestow on employees at all levels and whether they understand the consequences for certain behavior. Does everyone understand both the positive and negative consequences? Is it possible that you think you are giving a positive consequence, when in fact it is perceived as negative (power, FTEs, budget, and so on)?

Benefits of Working Together

There are several positive results from integrating human resources and marketing functions. The first is based on the belief that from both a real and a strategic standpoint, customer satisfaction is inextricably linked with employee satisfaction, especially in a service industry like health care. When you get all employees working together (by getting marketing and HR to work together) you are more likely to achieve organizational goals, your organization becomes more profitable, and you ensure its continued existence and your future employment.

A Profitable Venture

According to Cobb, Samuel, and Sexton (1998, p. 35), marketing and HR are as inextricably linked as customers and employees when you consider them from a strategic viewpoint. "First, a thorough knowledge of customers and the market should drive strategy. Second, strategy has to take into account not only the marketplace but also the organization, its capability and its employees. Third, the business strategy must have an accompanying, integrated HR strategy to ensure its implementation. Fourth, optimal execution of the business strategy depends on implementation of the HR strategy. Finally, monitoring and evaluating the effectiveness of the business strategy and the HR strategy are necessary, ongoing processes to provide feedback for continuous improvement."

A series of motivational experiments by Elton Mayo from 1927 to 1932 at Western Electric's Hawthorne Works in Cicero, Illinois, studied employees and managers at a real company and first uncovered the unmistakable relationship between worker attitudes and production (Rieger, 1995). Essentially, Mayo learned two things:

- Human beings regulate their involvement in and commitment to a given task or organization.
- The extent to which one does or does not fully contribute is governed more by attitude than by necessity, fear, or economic influence.

In their book *Contented Cows Give Better Milk*, Catlette and Hadden (1998, p. 7) say, "the only way for any organization to ensure its financial security is by creating satisfied, loyal customers. To the extent that the organization is at all labor-dependent, we propose that the principal requirement for operationalizing that aim is the creation of a satisfied, fully engaged workforce. In the main, our products and services, technology, methods, tools and strategies can all be copied. But it's not as easy to duplicate a focused, caring workforce. In the final analysis, 'people factors' are frequently the key source of competitive advantage."

Implementing programs, benefits, and policies that support employees in their jobs as well as in their family life will reap far more positive rewards in the future than any other single management effort. Employees who are well taken care of by their employer can better focus on taking care of customer needs.

Not everyone, however, can see the connection. One senior hospital executive was presented with a list of action items recommended by a customer relations council to achieve its customer relations program goals. The goals included such items as mandatory annual training, behavioral objectives, and several suggestions regarding improving employee morale such as recognition of positive performance and social activities. The senior executive crossed out the employee recognition and morale activities, saying these have "nothing to do with customer relations."

An Exchange of Information

The marketing department maintains an ongoing scan of the public's perception of your health care organization through patient satisfaction surveys, primary and secondary research, and feedback gained through involvement in community organizations. As such, the marketing staff is generally the keeper of the corporate image—but it should not be the sole image keeper. There are many other individuals within the organization who also are involved in community activities by virtue of their personal lives outside work.

The public perception of the organization needs to be shared among all levels of the organization—senior executives sharing "where we want to go" and all other employees providing feedback as to "how close we are to our goal."

Employees can provide incredibly good information simply by asking their friends, neighbors, and family members a few simple questions:

- Have you been a patient at the hospital I work for?
- What did you like about it?
- What can we do better?

The general public has an impression of the hospital as a provider of care but also as an employer. This information has a significant impact on human resources' ability to recruit qualified candidates, provide adequate benefits, and retain existing employees.

Another benefit of this exchange of information is that both departments will learn new skills that will help them within their primary functions. Human resources can reap additional benefits by learning more about the marketing of services, including the marketing of their own services to their internal customers. Marketing staff learn HR skills and expertise that will help them better define the organization to its various audiences.

Cross-Selling the Organization

When human resources and marketing departments are linked together, employees know not only the services provided by their clinical area, but the other services the hospital provides that could benefit the patient. Using employees to market other resources is a significant boost to the hospital's efforts.

Developing Core Competencies

Marketing staff can greatly assist HR staff in defining the type of employee that should be hired. The two functions together can create a powerful synergy, effective cross-trained teams, and a

service-oriented culture by defining the key competencies that support the core of their business, specific business initiatives or annual
objectives, customer service, productivity, and teamwork. Both
functions are familiar with the organization's goals. Marketing staff
know what the customer's expectations are. HR staff know how to
translate those expectations into key hiring criteria and performance development criteria. Together, they can work with operational   departments   to   change   functions,   redesign   job
responsibilities, and train staff to better perform their jobs to meet
customer expectations.

This can result in the development of realistic job previews,
structured interviews, interviewer training, and personality-based
assessment tools.

Satisfied Employees, Satisfied Customers

Attracting and retaining top performers is increasingly difficult for
health care providers. Creating an integrated approach to human
resources and marketing will give your organization an upper hand
in this effort by creating a workforce that

- Knows its goals and responsibilities
- Understands customer expectations
- Is given clear direction
- Is trained to do both the clinical and service aspects of the job
- Is provided with adequate support to perform the job

The end result is satisfied employees who no longer have to
focus on their own needs and can focus on the needs of their
patients and families. For your organization, the result is a reputation in the community as an employer of choice as well as a
provider of choice.

The HR department's job becomes easier because there are
more qualified candidates who apply for the few job openings that

become available through attrition or the many job openings that become available through growth.

The authors have, on more than one occasion, heard employees—and employers—say "well, nobody's irreplaceable" or "oh, well, good employees leave." The fact is good employees are not expendable or replaceable and there is no reason why they should have to leave the organization in order to progress in their profession. Sure, you can always find a "body" to replace an employee who leaves your hospital. But employees in whom you have invested significant resources in training, who have a strong knowledge of the organization, and who believe in and have a commitment to the mission, vision, and values of the organization are not easily and readily replaceable. And the real costs to the organization are significant in terms of time, quality, knowledge, and commitment.

That is why promotion of current employees is such a powerful tool for continued success. New ideas and energy can be introduced into the organization through hiring of new employees at entry levels. Through a planned employee development program, as described in Chapter 7, existing employees' skills can be developed so the employees become more valuable to the organization. Promoting existing employees into supervisory and management positions means that valuable training and development does not leave your organization and benefit some other facility.

The marketing department's job becomes easier because staff is able to focus on future patient needs, expansion of services, and targeting its message to specific audiences. The organization benefits because fewer resources (time and money) are being spent on advertising and external promotion and more on proactive steps to meet organizational goals.

Accreditation Issues

The standards for improving organization performance of the Joint Commission on Accreditation of Healthcare Organizations (Joint Commission) are another example of how a consolidated effort between human resources and marketing will reap rewards. According to the Joint Commission (1999), "Value in health care is the appropriate balance between good outcomes, excellent care and services, and costs. To add value to the care and services provided, organizations need to understand the relationship between perception of care, outcome and costs, and how processes carried out by the organization affect these three issues. An organization's performance of important functions significantly affects the quality and value of its services."

When marketing and HR work together, they create greater value for the organization and patients by understanding patient perceptions, outcomes, costs, and relationships. Employees not only know what the right things to do are, but they do them well. Patients and family members judge the value of their health care not only on whether or not they get well (the process and outcome), but also how on they were treated in the process.

In order to meet the Joint Commission's "Improving Organization Performance" standard, "activities are planned in a collaborative and interdisciplinary manner." Much of this standard speaks to patient satisfaction issues as well as clinical outcomes. What has an organization gained if the patient is cured, but is unhappy about the personal treatment received? The outcome does not stand alone.

Models for Working Together

Once any group of individuals within the organization (from senior leadership to staff employees within both departments) agree that there need to be greater linkages between HR and marketing, how do you do it? The answer is as individual as the organization. Each organization's set of circumstances—size, the personalities of the principals involved, the skill sets of the incumbents, and any other factor you can think of—is unique, and one model will not work for every organization.

For some organizations, the preferred model will require adding a new member to the executive leadership group (either HR or marketing—whoever is not currently present). For other organizations, the answer may be to have both functions report to the same senior executive—if he or she has the skills and expertise to manage both functional areas. For others, the best solution will be one integrated department combined under one talented person who has the vision to fully capitalize on the synergy that is possible. Yet others may choose to begin slowly and informally with special projects or teams working to meet common goals.

Many organizations have embraced the concept of organizational development (OD) created in industrial settings in the late 1950s and early 1960s. OD has various definitions ranging from a system of culture change or team building to a process that creates "better communication and coordination, improved organizational effectiveness leading to better business results, more satisfied employees and, ultimately, greater profitability" (Alexander, 1977, p. 134).

A broader definition is "a conscious, planned process of developing an organization's capabilities so that it can attain and sustain an optimum level of performance as measured by efficiency, effectiveness and health. Operationally, OD is a normative process of addressing the questions: 'Where are we?' 'Where do we want to be?' 'How do we get from where we are to where we want to be?' This process is undertaken by members of the organization using a variety of techniques" (McGill, 1977, p. 3).

Our definition of *organizational development* is developing the organization strategically through human resources, promotion, fund raising, and planning and linking all employees together to achieve organizational goals and create an environment of continuous improvement. This definition provides a broader description of OD and also allows for the integration of marketing and HR into that definition, for both of these functions ask the same questions within the context of the organization's goals. Most organizations having OD departments limit them to HR and training functions. With this broader definition of OD, it can encompass marketing, which seeks to develop the image of the organization and its continued viability, and fund raising, which seeks to develop financial support for a not-for-profit hospital.

Whichever model an organization chooses to use, realize that integration of two functions or departments is not an overnight process. The individuals within the departments will need to develop trust over time. The people committed to making this integration work—whether senior leadership or individual department employees—will have to maintain the commitment during difficult times. Especially in an organization in which there have been turf battles, the process will be slow in developing. It will be "more akin to a trek than a sprint" (Cobb, Samuel, and Sexton, 1998, p. 32).

Case Study: One Model for Integration at 1st Community Bank and Trust

In the summer of 1996 the board of directors of 1st Community Bank and Trust,* located just south of Indianapolis, began discussing the bank's growth and its need for a marketing professional. They also recognized that a human resources professional was a current and future need for the organization. The bank's need for two senior level executives led to discussions with area marketing and human resources professionals about linking the two functions. There seemed to be sufficient support and recognition that there was a link between the two functions and a job description was drafted.

To the bank president/CEO's mild surprise and great delight, there were several very qualified candidates who met the recruitment criteria for the position of vice president for human resources and marketing. After interviewing five candidates in the fall of 1997, the bank hired Don Goeb. At the time Goeb was hired, 1st Community had seven branches, $88 million in assets, fifty-nine

---

*This case study is based on an interview with Don Goeb, vice president, Human Resources and Marketing, 1st Community Bank and Trust, Greenwood, Indiana, October 21, 1998.

employees, and growth in the future in terms of both branches and assets. Goeb had his work cut out for him. In early 1999, the bank had nine branches, $120 million in assets, and more than sixty-five employees.

Luckily, Goeb's background was perfect for the position. He had worked in branch operations, human resources, and business development during his career, so he understood the importance of hiring the right people to fulfill customers' expectations and achieve the bank's operational goals.

Goeb was excited to integrate his various experiences. "One of my frustrations in HR was that I didn't have control of everything that I needed. Now that I'm in charge of both human resources and marketing, when I want to package my marketing plan, I can gear training to what we want to accomplish. I can have an impact on staffing of what we want to accomplish in marketing."

One example of how Goeb used his HR expertise to implement a marketing plan was an "officer call" program. The bank did not have a formalized program "for organizing branch managers to go into the community and educate people about 1st Community. It was my job to determine what we hoped to get out of an officer call program (we were already experiencing a lot of growth), who we wanted the officers to target, and, on the HR side, how we were going to be able to continue to keep the branch operational if we expect the branch managers to be out of the branch."

The plan required training the branch managers to place more focus on cross-training staff so they could handle certain issues when officers where not on site. Goeb also had to provide sales training to officers so they could effectively determine who to call on, what to say during the sales call, and what should happen after the initial call.

The program had mixed success after the first six months— something Goeb expected. "It's been extremely successful in some branches; there are training issues in others. It's a new concept, so it takes some time to get some 'old school' bankers to buy into the program."

Goeb credits the integration of HR and marketing to the program's viability. With more control and authority, he had the opportunity to deal with hurdles as they occurred. "In another organization, there likely wouldn't have been the training to support the program and it wouldn't have been as fully implemented," he said.

Another example of integrating the two functions is in the promotion of bank services—checking accounts, for instance. "I may have the brochures, posters, and ads ready but if the customer calls or walks in the door, are employees trained to answer questions and sell the program? If not, we've just wasted a lot of marketing dollars and we've lost opportunities. By being able to control the training as well as the marketing, I think we have a more successful checking program."

Training current employees is not Goeb's only challenge in integrating HR and marketing, especially in a competitive employment market (less than 2 percent unemployment).

"It gets more and more difficult to find the candidate you want," Goeb said. "I look at whether this person has the vision—is this person going to fit the culture and direction our board wants us to go in? There's a fantastic connection there. When I was in bank operations, I was looking at whether the person could do the job operationally. But now, I look at the whole process—dependability, operational ability, and can they help us get to where we want to go?"

With that type of integrated hiring approach, Goeb is able to better ensure that the employee who is hired is right for the job. Turnover at 1st Community is low, but everything is not always perfect. There are still relationships that go sour, as he puts it, so there are occasionally avoidable losses of good, qualified employees.

Goeb realizes that the size advantage of 1st Community has helped with the integration of the two functions. "The larger the bank organization, the more bureaucratic you tend to have to be, " he said. "Any time you add another person, you throw a new personality into the mix, each with his or her own agenda. This [integrating HR and marketing] is such an obvious tie together. I was excited and nervous about biting off more than I could chew when I started. But it's worked out very well. I had done each of the jobs independently, so putting them together was just natural."

There continue to be challenges in Goeb's position, but not necessarily as a result of the combined responsibilities. With bank growth come new challenges: "We keep growing. When I started, we just went over the magic number of fifty employees, which opens up compliance issues and reporting and documentation requirements. I think I'm about ready for an HR assistant who can make sure benefits are in line and being promoted to employees."

References

Alexander, C. P. "The Perils and Pitfalls of an OD Effort." In D. F. Van Eynde, J. C. Hoy, and D. C. Van Eynde (eds.), *Organization Development Classics*. San Francisco: Jossey-Bass, 1977.

American Hospital Association. "Reality √: Public Perceptions of Health Care and Hospitals." Chicago: American Hospital Association, 1996.

American Hospital Association. "Reality √ II: More Public Perceptions of Health Care and Hospitals." Chicago: American Hospital Association, 1997–1998.

Catlette, B., and Hadden, R. *Contented Cows Give Better Milk*. Germantown, Tenn.: Saltillo Press, 1998.

Cobb, J. C., Samuel, C. J., and Sexton, M. W. "Alignment and Strategic Change: A Challenge for Marketing and Human Resources." *Leadership & Organization Development Journal*, 1998, 19(1), 32–43.

Health Forum, Arthur Andersen, and DYG. *Leadership for a Healthy 21st Century*. Chicago: Health Forum, 1999.

Hequet, M. "Beyond Dollars." *Training*, Mar. 1996.

Joint Commission on Accreditation of Healthcare Organizations. *CAMH Refreshed Core*. Oakbrook Terrace, Ill.: Joint Commission on Accreditation of Healthcare Organizations, Jan. 1999.

McGill, M. *Organization Development for Operating Managers*. New York: AMACOM, 1977.

Rieger, B. "Lessons in Productivity and People." *Training and Development*, 1995, 49(10), 56.

Russell, L. "Painting the Future Picture: Changing an Organization by Moving Beyond Its Comfort Zone." *Health Forum Journal*, Jan./Feb. 1999.

Chapter Five

Recruiting and Motivating a Changing Workforce

Traditional functions of human resources departments include, among others, creating job descriptions, developing performance appraisal systems, and interviewing prospective employees. Defining which employees are right for an organization can be accomplished more effectively by adding some creative variations to these traditional functions. The first step in hiring the right people is to staff the human resources department with people who have the qualities that are deemed important in employees to serve as role models. These are often the first contact employees have with the organization and they continue to be employee advocates (Rosenbluth and Peters, 1998, p. 64).

While an organization is appealing to consumers in a defined geographic area, it is also appealing to the same population base for potential employees. The wording and appearance of advertisements may provide an individual's first impression of an organization. It may be beneficial to integrate the efforts of the people responsible for advertising services and those responsible for ads recruiting employees. In practice, however, some marketing and human resources departments are "not only not integrated but in fact rarely talk to each other" (Cobb, Samuel, and Sexton, 1998, p. 32). This chapter will explore some of the ways health care organizations can expand traditional human resources practices to market their organizations more effectively to potential employees.

The Changing Workplace

Trends in the workforce have created some difficulty in finding the right employees. The net addition to the workforce, defined as the number of people coming into the workforce minus the number that leave, has moved from 3 percent in the 1970s and 1980s to approximately 1 percent in 1998 (Losey, 1998, p. 27). This trend creates more competition for organizations trying to attract and retain the best workers. Companies are working harder to sell their organization to prospective employees. Increasingly, prospective employees are interviewing the companies as much as the companies are interviewing them (Lee, 1997, p. 28).

As a result of the decrease in number of qualified workers entering the workforce, potential employees are becoming better informed about ways to be wise consumers as they search for the right employer. Prospective employees are coached by career counselors to ask questions during interviews to determine the level of commitment an organization has to its vision and mission. Job seekers are often encouraged to investigate the organizational priorities of the potential employer before making a decision about accepting a position. They may talk to friends who work for the organization, check the Internet for information, or request information from the human resources department describing the organization's philosophy, mission, values, and so on to be sure they are considering a company whose policies will fit their personal values. Generation X employees in particular are more likely to request detailed information about multiple aspects of a job and a company's policies before accepting a position in a company (Kupperschmidt, 1998, p. 40).

Recruitment and retention are not mutually exclusive activities. If employees are getting the things they value from a workplace, they become tangible advertisements for the organization. If the employer is offering the kinds of benefits to employees that make them happy in their work, the organization becomes known as one of the places where people want to work. This is one example of word-of-mouth advertising at its best. Happy employees not only lead to happy customers; they also have the ability to recruit additional happy employees.

Worker Expectations

Health care organizations have a dual role in appealing to workers. People who choose clinical health care careers may have some very different motivations for choosing their work compared with those in such service industries as food services, accounting, or information services. Attracting the best workers to such a diverse workplace as a health care facility requires an understanding of what motivates workers in general and also an understanding of what motivates workers who are in clinical health care roles.

A study of 3,000 workers conducted by the Families and Work Institute indicated that learning opportunities increase worker loyalty to the company. The study highlighted a total of five components that make up how workers measure job quality:

- Autonomy
- Learning opportunities
- Meaningfulness of the job
- Job security
- Personal opportunities for advancement.

All of these factors were "positively related to employee retention and loyalty to the company" (Jacobson, 1998, p. 16).

To understand why an employee chooses a particular organization, it may be helpful to understand why employees leave organizations. Michael Losey, president and CEO of the Society for Human Resource Management, has cited the top three reasons people leave organizations:

1. They see a better opportunity and better benefits.
2. They are not sure of their career potential where they are.

3. They do not feel appreciated in their current company (Losey, 1998, p. 27).

A comparison of the two lists above—factors that employees identify with job quality and the reasons employees leave organizations—sheds some light on the priorities of employees. The common themes in these lists are the issues employers need to address if they want to find and hire the best workers. It may not be feasible to develop plans to address all of the issues cited, but the information provides an opportunity for organizations to capitalize on the areas in which they have particular strengths.

Recruiting Students

Many health care organizations provide special programs to recruit students in nursing and other clinical preparation programs with the hope of enticing those individuals to remain in the organization as employees once they have completed their formal training. Student technician positions allow students to gain valuable work experience prior to graduating and also provide them with an excellent opportunity to assess the positive and negative aspects of a workplace. They are working alongside employees who are often willing to share not only technical knowledge, but also their own personal feelings about the employer and the unwritten rules or the culture of the organization. These activities can begin the process of socializing workers into the organization.

Health care organizations often provide students with a shorter orientation program than that provided to new employees because students tend to be employed for a limited time and therefore need only the essential information about minimum safety requirements. Providing the same full-scale orientation offered employees would not be cost effective; however, an orientation that goes beyond the basic safety information would make a positive statement to the students about the value the organization places on people.

Students as young as middle-school or high-school age are increasingly becoming involved in school-to-work programs in which they have opportunities to shadow an employee for several days or weeks to learn about the day-to-day responsibilities of a particular job. Students at this age may not be eligible for employment, but the value of word-of-mouth advertising about their experiences should not be overlooked. Students share their experiences with friends, neighbors, and family members who may have had little or no previous contact with the organization. Hospitals are often associated with illness and therefore perceived as places to be avoided. Students of various ages are in a position to learn about some of the more positive aspects of health care and pass along those positive images to others.

Recruiting Experienced Workers

Recruitment devices for highly skilled jobs in health care include creative incentives. Some health care organizations are offering cash sign-on bonuses as an incentive to RNs and other clinical specialists, and others are appealing to lifestyle issues to get their attention. Workplaces are marketing their family-friendly policies to appeal to potential employees. Some hospitals are offering other creative incentives including

- Free child care for a designated period
- Free house cleaning services for up to one year
- Payoff of student loans
- Traditional sign-on cash bonuses

A recruiting brochure for a rural hospital near a large metropolitan city was recently developed and mailed to the homes of RNs in a defined geographic area. The brochure was designed to appeal to people who would appreciate the slower pace of a rural setting. The hospital is located within commuting distance of the large city with multiple teaching hospitals for nurses and other health care workers to choose from. The subtle message is that a more relaxed work environment exists in the rural hospital.

These examples illustrate the need for marketing and human resources departments within an organization to collaborate in determining the priorities of prospective employees and the most efficient ways to convey the organization's values. It is worth noting that financial issues were not explicitly mentioned in the previous list of factors employees value in a job or the reasons employees leave a job. Increasingly, workers cite issues of personal growth; yet the financial bonuses continue to be used as a recruiting tool to attract health care workers. Data from exit interviews may reveal important information about how particular organizations can change to meet the shifting priorities of the workforce.

If financial issues are not a strong consideration in employees' career decisions, it may be wise for employers to be even more creative with incentives and look beyond the traditional sign-on bonus. A survey conducted by the outplacement firm Lee Hecht Harrison indicated that turnover rates actually increased in companies where pay increases were the only incentive. According to Cathy Kennedy, vice president for Lee Hecht Harrison, it takes more than money to keep the best employees in a company. While some other company can always outbid an employer, it may be more difficult to compete with a reputation of having an exceptional work environment (Leonard, 1998, p. 22).

Recruiting the Right People

People who choose health careers are often driven by the desire to be of service or make a difference in the lives of others. They cite such attractions as the ability to continue learning, more job security than other careers, and flexibility. The health care industry sometimes has difficulty in defining and measuring attitudes that may be inherent in the people who choose a profession that would allow them to help others.

Human resources professionals, training specialists, and marketing professionals may all be involved in efforts to build the soft skills of the workforce. Technical skills are easily defined and measured by competency checklists and written procedures and protocols. Skills related to customer service, teamwork, pride, and other attitudes are more difficult to quantify.

When health care organizations recruit workers, they often use data on local and sometimes national employment trends. These data may be helpful in identifying where the qualified workers are. However, an important follow-up activity is assessing the attitudes and motivations of the workers they are trying to recruit. In their effort to get open positions filled, managers may either give low priority to assessing the attitude or personality of the prospective employee or rely on training and development activities and the performance appraisal process to motivate the employee to demonstrate desired behaviors.

The nature of the work that is carried out in health care organizations makes competence in technical skills a priority. Organizations that are trying to keep up with shortages of specific kinds of skilled workers and at the same time attract entry-level employees in other areas of the organization may believe it is not feasible to get both technical competence and good attitude in all employees. Organizations will sometimes resort to the "warm body syndrome" familiar to many health care workers. Managers who see their staff stretched to their limits may overlook personality issues if the prospective employee has the right technical skills and credentials.

Health care organizations can benefit by observing other industries to find ways to improve a variety of their practices. Organizations that have committed to a formalized continuous improvement philosophy are especially likely to benchmark with other kinds of industries. In some industries, the primary attribute sought in new employees is the right attitude. One particular company has identified a unique approach to hiring the right employees. Hal Rosenbluth is the owner of a multimillion dollar travel company and author of the book, *The Customer Comes Second*. The one quality he deems most important when interviewing prospective employees is whether the person is nice. His philosophy is to hire nice people, treat them and train them well, and give them the best technology to be successful in their jobs (Henkoff, 1994, p. 120).

In the highly technical health care industry, some professionals who are involved in the hiring process might question the need to hire nice people as workers. However, research indicates that consumer expectations of health care services are based on relationships. In a competitive market, organizations cannot afford to think of appropriate attitudes, personalities, or motivations as optional qualities to expect in employees.

The importance of behaviors was quantified in a study of the reasons 200 diverse companies fired people from their jobs. The study indicated that people are usually fired because of a personality issue, not because of poor performance. The study showed that 70 percent of those fired could not get along with others in the organization (Basile, 1998, p. 21).

Measuring Behavior

Although it may be difficult to measure personality traits, it is essential to implement policies and practices that will attempt to improve the way these traits are measured, both in job descriptions and in performance appraisals. If health care leaders are to be successful in responding to the expectations of both employees and customers, they will need to develop creative strategies to convey and demonstrate their core values to both of these groups. Many health care organizations have adopted a continuous improvement philosophy, whether by internal design or in response to the changing expectations of organizations such as the Joint Commission.

The organization may choose to define expectations of employee behavior based on the organization's quality improvement processes, mission, or values or a combination of all of these factors. Some organizations have placed a high priority on their mission or values by making consistent statements of expectations in every job description throughout the organization. Following the initial statements are the detailed responsibilities for the individual job. Prospective employees benefit by seeing detailed expectations clearly defined in job descriptions. These should also include behavioral expectations, allowing individuals to decide whether their values match those of the organization. Detailed descriptions of expectations decrease the chance of disappointment in the initial weeks or even days of orientation.

Performance Appraisals

One of the least favorite responsibilities of many managers and supervisors in health care is providing written performance appraisals and discussions with employees. Measuring and defining attitudes, values, and other soft skills can be difficult and frustrating for both the evaluator and the person receiving the evaluation. Various approaches discussed in Chapter 7 are available to make this process more beneficial for both the employee and the organization.

Behavioral Objectives

In an effort to reduce employee turnover at Johnson Memorial Hospital, a 165-bed county hospital located in Franklin, Indiana, a committee was formed to recommend actions that might decrease turnover and improve employee morale. Based on one of the recommendations, an educational workshop for all employees was planned. The goal of the workshop was to improve communication and customer service skills. The all-day workshop was presented numerous times throughout the year so that all employees could be scheduled to attend.

Specific competency criteria for each position in the organization were developed. The competencies were created jointly by managers and employees and are designed to be individualized to each employee's job. Lists of specific skills that will move an employee to the next level on the competency scale correspond with increases in the wage scale. These competencies provide employees with specific, measurable criteria for improving their performance. Defined behavioral expectations are consistent with the messages the employees hear in the educational workshop focusing on communication and customer service skills.

Rewards and Recognition

Because behavior that is rewarded tends to be repeated, several recognition awards were also implemented at Johnson Memorial. A few traditional awards, such as employee of the month, were already in place. Additional awards were developed to encourage employees to take the extra steps to model behaviors related to teamwork, leadership, or customer service. Figure 5.1 provides a brief description of the awards.

Profiles of award recipients are included in the hospital's internal and external newsletters. This publicity further rewards the employees with public recognition of their accomplishments and communicates the organization's values to the community.

Diversity Issues

The Americans with Disabilities Act has focused attention on issues of diversity, and the Joint Commission has increased its emphasis on diversity awareness in its standards. An example is a standard in the patient and family education chapter of the guidelines, which states that organizations are responsible for identifying any religious or cultural barriers that could interfere with the patient's ability to learn the information that will be shared during his or her hospital stay.

Educational programs that highlight diversity issues are often presented within health care organizations or in conjunction with professional seminars. Many of these presentations focus on diversity in the community served or in the patient population.

Figure 5.1. Johnson Memorial Hospital Award Programs.

Have you become confused about the different award programs that the hospital is sponsoring to show appreciation for employee efforts? Well apparently, you are not alone. Human Resources has compiled the following information to help you understand each of these programs better and how you and your coworkers may be affected. Keep in mind that except for the SHARE Program, anyone can nominate another staff member for one of these awards. In the case of Employee of the Month and the Key Contributor Award, you can even nominate yourself.

Program	Sponsor	Eligibility	How Often	Particulars
Above & Beyond Award	T.E.A.M. Committee	All employees	Twice a year	• Designed to give hospitalwide recognition and reinforce behavior that exceeds expectations as it relates to teamwork, leadership, and customer service. • Nominations are to be sent to the T.E.A.M. Committee. • Winners attend a reception held in their honor and receive an engraved plaque and gift certificate. Their names are also placed on a group plaque, which hangs outside the cafeteria. Winners are announced in *Hospital Happenings* and *Focus on Health*.
Employee of the Month	Employee Relations Council	All employees	Once a month, effective January 1998	• Recognizes individuals who have exhibited a positive attitude toward their coworkers and very good customer service skills, perform their job well, and may have thought of some cost savings ideas.

(Continued)

Figure 5.1. Continued.

Program	Sponsor	Eligibility	How Often	Particulars
				• Nominations are to be sent to the Employee Relations Council *via* the Human Resources Department. • Winners receive their name on a plaque, an announcement in *Hospital Happenings*, and a gift certificate for dinner, Merry Maids service, etc., or a pair of pro sports tickets.
Key Contributor Award	Key Contributor Award Committee	Nonmanagement employees	Monthly	• Recognizes individuals who have gone above and beyond their regular duties to identify and implement a program that results in cost reduction, revenue enhancement, improved quality, improved productivity, and/or improved customer satisfaction (internal and/or external customers). • Nominations are to be sent to the Key Contributor Award Committee *via* the Human Resources Department. • Winners receive a cash award generally ranging from $500 to $1,000.

| Risky Business Award | T.E.A.M. Committee | All employees | Twice a year | • Recognizes staff who have taken some type of risk, such as a new idea to change a process.
• Nominations are to be sent to the T.E.A.M. Committee.
• Winners receive a gift certificate. |
| SHARE Program | SHARE Committee/ Hospital Board of Trustees | Nonmanagement employees (see details in far right column) | Annually, usually paid in March or April of the following year | • Employee must be regularly scheduled full- or part-time and employed prior to 10/1 of the plan year to be eligible.
• All eligible employees will share in the positive financial performance of the hospital to a maximum of 30% of the excess revenue if 100% of the SHARE goals are met for that year. |

Education on diversity issues within the health care worker population is important in promoting teamwork and cooperation in an industry that has demanding work responsibilities. There are many factors to be considered in understanding the various elements of diversity and their impact on the workplace. Companies may go to great lengths to recruit a diverse workforce and ultimately lose workers because the culture of the organization does not truly support them (Austin, 1998, p. 21).

One example of a diversity issue that affects the workplace is employee age. Understanding the values and motivations of various generations can provide valuable information about policies and structures that support employees' efforts to produce high-quality work.

Generation X

Defined as the group of workers born between approximately 1961 and 1981, this group is gaining increased attention as more of its members move into the workplace. Most descriptions of characteristics describing Generation X begin with the negative characteristics. These include a short attention span, lack of a work ethic, and a self-absorbed attitude. Some of the positive characteristics associated with this group include pragmatism and resourcefulness. Many people from this generation moved around during their childhood years as a result of changes in their parents' jobs or marital status. Many have a great deal of experience making decisions on their own. This generation is comfortable with change because it has been a way of life.

Since Generation X is so comfortable with change, workers in this group are more likely than others to change jobs if they believe their professional needs are not being met. Individuals in this group tend to want specific, measurable goals and feedback in the workplace. They want the work environment to have values that match their own. Continuous learning is important to them from the standpoint that it keeps them challenged and increases their marketability in the workplace (Kupperschmidt, 1998, p. 42).

Baby Boomers

Baby boomers are traditionally defined as the group of people born between approximately 1946 and 1964. Baby boomers have observed many changes in society and as a result are prone to questioning or challenging existing structures in society in general as well as in the workplace. Individuals in this group are sometimes characterized as looking out for number one. They tend to be futuristic thinkers because they like to explore options and experiment with new ideas.

Baby boomers place a high premium on quality of life and quality of work. They expect to have fun at work by nature of their tendency to question existing ideas and experiment with new ways of thinking. They value freedom and self-expression as components of their jobs.

Traditionalists

This title is not as quickly recognized as the more publicized Generation X and baby boomers. The individuals in this group actually cross over the generation boundaries of baby boomers and the generation just prior to that era. Traditionalists include people whose values were shaped in the 1920s to the 1950s. They are accepting of rank order, loyal to institutions, and much of their self-identity is tied to their work. They believe in solving their own problems and value stability in relationships.

Individuals who have traditionalist values are often the ones who have been in an organization for fifteen years or more. They seek meaningful involvement in the organization; consequently, they tend to be loyal employees. These employees do not adjust well to the concept of cross-training or combining tasks (adapted from Hamilton, 1998; Blalock and Hobart, 1998).

These descriptions provide a brief example of the variety of needs and expectations of various generations of workers. Examples of additional diversity issues include those related to race, gender, and lifestyle. Researching and understanding diversity issues require a significant commitment of time and resources.

One method of prioritizing which elements of diversity are most significant to address in a particular organization is to identify the employee population by demographics. The workforce can be profiled by five major categories:

- Age
- Gender
- Ethnicity
- Education
- Disability (Jamieson and O'Mara, 1991, pp. 179–181)

Creating a matrix detailing numbers of employees in identified categories can be helpful in quantifying the prevalence of specific groups within the workforce. Other factors that may be considered include years of work experience and marital and parental status.

Once the data have been collected, it is essential to gather information directly from the employees to help interpret the data. Biases and assumptions from the data can be inaccurate unless the people directly involved are consulted to determine what the data mean to them. Examples of ways to get information from employees include

- Discussion groups representing large segments of the workforce
- Advisory groups with special expertise
- Task forces for special studies
- Surveys of all or a sample of employees
- Individual interviews

This follow-up approach helps to ensure analysis of needs and values that is descriptive, not judgmental (Jamieson and O'Mara, 1991, pp. 179–181).

Work and Personal Issues

A study conducted by Mercer (1996) investigated the importance of addressing personal and diversity issues of employees. The survey included more than 800 various types of organizations throughout the country. Most companies (86 percent) agree that personal and diversity issues must be addressed if they are to remain competitive. In response to the changing demographics of the workforce, employers recognize the importance of programs that meet employees' personal as well as work needs in their recruitment efforts. The three programs they identified as most important include

- Flexible scheduling
- Paid time off
- Child care

Flexible scheduling may encompass a number of creative scheduling options, including job sharing, compressed work weeks, working from home, increased options for maternity and paternity leaves, and programs to help balance the needs of the family. A variety of employers define the core component of flexible scheduling as a system that gives employees more control over their own time. The specific policies for an organization ideally are influenced by the demographics of the workers in that organization.

Companies are reevaluating their paid time off policies in an attempt to address the changing demographics of the workforce. Employees who are caring for children or elderly parents (or sometimes both) need paid time off policies that allow them flexibility to take care of their families as well as themselves.

Child care assistance programs are expanding to include services that go beyond on-site day care centers. Other programs for children include sick child care, summer camp programs, after-school programs, and flexible spending accounts to improve the ability of parents to financially manage these services (adapted from Mercer, 1996).

Keeping Employees Motivated in Difficult Times

Many of the trends described up to this point have prompted employers to find creative ways to recruit new workers to their organizations. At the same time, employers must search for ways to keep their current workforce motivated under the unpleasant circumstances of working harder to make up for the gaps created by open positions. While employees are trying to adjust to the ongoing stress of working harder with fewer available resources, personal stresses continue to compound.

The Mercer (1996) study also found that employee assistance plans (EAPs) were offered by more than three-quarters of the respondents to the survey. Other counseling programs reported by the respondents include, among others: stress management, grief/terminal illness counseling, child care and elder care counseling, and skills assessment counseling. Employers are attempting to implement programs that will help employees balance their life at work with their life at home.

The strongest competitor an employer has for a particular employee may not be a similar employer who will pay more or provide better benefits—it may be the family or the free time of the employee. Workers may have children and elderly parents to care for. Coping with a chronic illness or death of a parent or safety concerns about children who may be home alone take a toll on employees, who may be preoccupied at work with these family concerns.

The American Hospice Association has created a booklet *Grief at Work* to be used as a tool to help managers understand and cope with absenteeism and performance issues caused by the many people in the workplace who are in one of the stages of grief. A regular feature in many EAP publications is information on coping with various kinds of stress, and there is a variety of literature and seminars that deal with issues of stress and coping in the workplace.

Implications of Health Promotion for the Workplace

Hospitals and health care organizations are increasingly addressing issues of health promotion. As managed care continues to expand in communities, it is in the best interest of health care providers to invest more resources into activities that promote health and wellness. The economic incentives of keeping individual health plan subscribers from becoming inpatients, combined with increasingly knowledgeable health care consumers requesting wellness services, are making prevention of illness a necessity, rather than a luxury.

Expanding the focus of services to include health promotion has an impact on the workforce. Many businesses, including health care organizations, are providing fitness centers, regularly scheduled wellness screenings, and incentives for participating in wellness programs. If health care organizations try to implement health promotion services in the community but fail to carry that philosophy over to their own employees, the inconsistency will compromise their perceived commitment to those services.

Looking out for the health and well-being of employees is an example of one way organizations can literally treat employees as customers. Ideally, companies should show the same concern for satisfying the needs of employees as the employees are expected to show when dealing with external customers. The benefit for employers is promoting a workforce that chooses healthy behaviors, which could ultimately both decrease absenteeism resulting from illness and increase satisfaction with the workplace.

According to Dr. Brian Wong, partner and worldwide director of health care strategy for Arthur Andersen, " . . . the business of healthcare may very well be about the business of relationships, relationships that support and enhance the health and well-being of not just the organization itself, but of the employees, and the consumers and communities they serve" (Mycek, 1998, p. 30).

Case Study: Following the Disney Model at University of Chicago Hospitals

In recent years, the University of Chicago Hospitals system* has made substantial commitments to improvements in several key areas. These include fine-tuning hiring practices, establishing an educational academy to educate staff at all levels, and creating an atmosphere that values employees and promotes respect for patients and colleagues. One indication of the success of its efforts is its recognition by *U.S. News and World Report* in 1998 as one of America's best hospitals.

The organization also received the "Mouseker Award" in 1998. This award, presented by Disney, recognized the hospital system's efforts to provide outstanding service to patients and customers. Many of Disney's principles of outstanding service have been incorporated into the system's policies and practices. In addition, it has created a partnership with Disney for organizational training programs. Disney Institute representatives videotaped examples of excellence in hiring, training, and patient care at multiple sites in the hospital system in order to use the footage in training sessions for other health care organizations.

University of Chicago Hospitals hires and trains people with service in mind. Hospital leaders have systems in place to measure service, give feedback to employees, and celebrate successes.

Benchmark studies of other service leaders, including the Ritz-Carlton Hotel, Motorola, and Avis also provided valuable informa-

---

*Documents used with permission of University of Chicago Hospitals, including *UCH Academy Quarterly*, summer/fall 1998; and "Launching an Organizational Change Strategy for Building Cultural Competence," a presentation by Steven H. Lipstein, executive vice president, and JoAnn M. Shaw, vice president and chief human resources officer, University of Chicago Hospitals and Health System, June 22, 1999.

tion to the system's leaders about what makes these organizations so successful in providing customer service.

Hiring Practices

The system's "Right Person . . . Right Role" process is designed to make sure the best person for a job is in that particular job. Before completing an application form, job candidates watch a video describing the mission, values, and expectations of the organization. This preview helps candidates decide for themselves whether they believe they would fit in the culture of the organization. Interview questions are behaviorally based to provide an assessment of the candidate's cultural competence. An important theme in University of Chicago Hospitals' strategic plan is providing for the needs of a diverse population of customers. Interview questions include queries to directly assess the cultural competence of candidates, particularly those in leadership roles. Examples of cultural assessment interview questions include:

- "Please describe your past experiences in working in a culturally diverse work environment."
- "In what ways have you demonstrated your commitment to building an inclusive work environment that values diversity?"

Cultural competence continues to be reinforced in a variety of ways following the initial interview. Staff development programs are constructed using the theme of cultural competence. A diversity action council acts as an advisory group to continue the focus on cultural diversity, bringing awareness to the forefront in the day-to-day operations of the organization. Cultural competence is also incorporated into individual employee performance appraisals. Exit interviews provide an additional opportunity for the organization to assess its effectiveness in promoting cultural diversity.

Learning Academy—Continuing Education

Once the right people are placed in the right jobs, the organization is committed to helping employees be a part of the best workforce possible by providing multiple educational opportunities.

The UCH Academy was created to prepare workers for future challenges through formal education programs, which include a variety of courses designed to meet the learning needs of a diverse employee population. Some of the courses offered include: a graduation equivalency diploma course, English as a second language, management training, and interpersonal communications. Courses are intended to help employees expand their opportunities for personal and professional growth. Some courses are taught directly through the UCH Academy, while others are coordinated through local colleges and universities.

In addition to providing information to participants, the courses also promote strategies for working together with others to solve problems or work more efficiently. A senior executive and member of the group that designed the original concept for the UCH Academy refers to it as "the most significant gift" that the University of Chicago Hospitals ever gave to its employees.

Summary

Health care leaders rely on data to measure the overall success of their organizations. Measurement of the success of customer service, cultural competence, and other skills that may be considered soft skills is also necessary for success.

These skills are perceived by many health care leaders to contribute to meeting organizational goals. In a climate of cost cutting, it becomes vitally important to move beyond a broad perception of value to quantifiable measures of success. One such measure is employee turnover. The University of Chicago Hospitals' employee retention rate improved from 74 percent to 82 percent over a six-year period. Just as preventive health practices are becoming more widely recognized for their actual cost-saving features, reduction in turnover rates is becoming more widely recognized as a valid measure of success of employee training and development activities. The University of Chicago Hospitals system demonstrates the value of a true service commitment to both internal and external customers.

References

Austin, N. K. "Killing Employees with Kindness." *Working Woman*, Jan. 1998.

Basile, F. "Avoid the Ax by Being Competent and Likable." *Indianapolis Business Journal*, June 15–21, 1998.

Blalock, T., and Hobart, A. "Bridging the Gap: Teaching Across the Lifespan." Conference presentation, "Making the Most Out of the Complex Health Care Environment," Cary, N.C., Oct. 21–23, 1998.

Cobb, J. C., Samuel, C. J., and Sexton, M. W. "Alignment and Strategic Change: A Challenge for Marketing and Human Resources." *Leadership & Organization Development Journal*, 1998, 19(1), 32–43.

Hamilton, L. "Living by Values in the Workplace." Conference presentation, "Making the Most Out of the Complex Health Care Environment," Cary, N.C., Oct. 21–23, 1998.

Henkoff, R. "Finding, Training, and Keeping the Best Service Workers." *Fortune*, Oct. 3, 1994.

Jacobson, D. "Nonstop Learning, Dead-End Jobs." *Training*, Sept. 1998, 35(9).

Jamieson, D., and O'Mara, J. *Managing Workforce 2000: Gaining the Diversity Advantage*. San Francisco: Jossey-Bass, 1991.

Kupperschmidt, B. R. "Understanding Generation X Employees." *Journal of Nursing Administration*, Dec. 1998, 28(12).

Lee, C. "The Hunt for Skilled Workers." *Training*, Dec. 1997, 34(12).

Leonard, B. "Continuing High Turnover Frustrating Employees." *H.R. Magazine*, Oct. 1998, 43(11).

Losey, D. *Washington Business Journal*, July 3, 1998, 27(8).

Mercer, W. M. Work/Life and Diversity Initiatives Benchmarking Survey. New York: Mercer, 1996.

Mycek, S. "Leadership for a Healthy 21st Century." *Healthcare Forum Journal*, July/Aug. 1998.

Rosenbluth, H. F., and Peters, D. M. *Good Company: Caring as Fiercely as You Compete*. Reading, Mass.: Addison-Wesley, 1998.

Chapter Six

Hiring the Right People

Once an organization has committed to the ongoing process of defining the characteristics that will make it successful, it has a vested interest in hiring the people who will continue to promote the values it defines. Without determining the characteristics of the right kind of employees, it is nearly impossible to know which candidate is the right one. The cost of a bad hiring decision has been estimated to be 30 percent of the employee's first year of potential earnings. Other indirect costs include the cost of

- Training a replacement
- Potentially losing customers
- Classified advertising
- Lower productivity
- Travel expenses
- Possible unemployment compensation claim
- Low morale (Hacker, 1996, p. xii)

Organizations may rely on a number of employees to be involved in the interviewing process. Anyone who is involved in this function should be aware of basic guidelines for interviewing, not only for legal purposes but also to be able to make informed decisions about job candidates. This chapter will review some guidelines for recruiting and interviewing the best employees possible by incorporating the values of the organization in the messages prospective employees receive.

Demographic Shifts in the Workplace

Understanding the shifts occurring in workforce demographics will help employers understand the priorities of current and future employees. Demographic data can help provide information about locating the right people and getting recruiting information to them in a way that encourages them to find out more about the organization.

As the number of middle-aged workers in the workforce continues to increase, the number of workers aged sixteen to twenty-four continues to decline. The younger workers are traditionally sought to fill entry-level positions. Advances in health care and increased priority on wellness programs are keeping people in the workforce for a longer period of time. Following are some of the possible implications for the workforce as a result of these demographic shifts:

- Younger employees will manage older employees in increasing numbers.
- Older workers will probably be less willing than younger workers to relocate because of ties to their community.
- There will be increased emphasis on policies related to wellness, family, and dependent care.
- Reward systems will shift to include perks such as increased time off or sabbaticals instead of traditional salary increases.
- Motivations for working will shift as workers get older. The kind of work that was viewed as challenging at one time may seem very different as employees get older (Jamieson and O'Mara, 1991, pp. 16–17).

Characteristics of Fulfilling Work

A variety of research indicates that most people want to accomplish more in their work than simply making a living. Work that is fulfilling allows people to be creative and flexible. It provides people with a sense of pride in their accomplishments and recognition from others for their efforts. Employees want to be treated fairly and to be able to achieve a balance between their work and personal life. They will not be able to achieve these goals unless the employer understands their priorities and creates a culture that supports them.

A Gallup study identified twelve worker beliefs that play a role in a profitable, productive workplace. These beliefs are:

1. I know what is expected of me at work.

2. I have the materials and equipment I need to do my work right.

3. At work, I have the opportunity to do what I do best every day.

4. In the last seven days, I have received recognition or praise for doing good work.

5. My supervisor or someone else at work seems to care about me as a person.

6. There is someone at work who encourages my development.

7. In the past six months, someone at work has talked to me about my progress.

8. At work, my opinions seem to count.

9. The mission and purpose of my company make me feel my job is important.

10. My fellow employees are committed to doing high-quality work.

11. I have a best friend at work.

12. This last year, I have had opportunities at work to learn and grow (Micco, 1998, p. 16).

Characteristics of the Right Employees for Your Organization

Health care organizations are increasingly involving their employees in a variety of community activities. These efforts are often linked to community health programs; but community involvement can also enhance an organization's recruitment and hiring efforts in a positive way. An example of a community program that is rapidly expanding in the Indianapolis area is the School-to-Work program.

Following a seminar on preparing students for the workforce, the Franklin Community School Corporation's school-to-work program conducted a series of focus group interviews throughout the community. The focus groups were composed of representatives from a wide variety of businesses and industries, including health care, construction, legal services, social services, manufacturing, agriculture, and media, to name a few. The members of the focus groups were asked two questions:

1. What should students know and be able to do by the time they graduate?
2. What skills do they need in order to succeed in a technology-based society of the future?

The responses of the various groups were recorded and later divided into categories. The number of skills that could be categorized as "social" or "life" skills outnumbered academic, technical, and workplace skills combined. Some of the recommended academic skills include:

- Effective oral and written communication skills
- Technical reading and writing
- Math skills: addition, subtraction, multiplication, division, and so on
- Knowledge of how and when to apply math skills
- Ability to alphabetize
- Basic science
- Foreign language
- Appreciation of the arts

A partial list of the recommended social or life skills includes:

- Motivation, initiative, being an encourager
- Pride in self and appearance
- Sense of ownership, responsibility, and reliability
- Desire to learn
- Anger control
- Social responsibility
- Customer service skills
- Voluntary community service
- Setting goals annually
- Lifelong learning
- Ability to work as a team member
- Willingness to accept accountability for decisions
- Flexibility
- Pride in job
- Ability to manage time
- Safety awareness

The findings of this project have implications for health care organizations. They need to

- Be aware of research indicating that consumers, assuming technical competence in health care workers, are more concerned with their social skills
- Reinforce the need for health care workers to role model appropriate attitudes and behavior for students and others who come in contact with the hospital
- Provide an opportunity for the local hospital to set an example in the community by incorporating behavioral components into the hiring and performance appraisal systems

Recruitment

Many health care organizations offer incentives such as sign-on bonuses, flexible scheduling, and tuition reimbursement in an effort to attract employees. Becoming an organization that is widely recognized as a good place to work requires additional incentives in the form of policies and practices that will support employees' needs for recognition and personal development. This is an area where employers need to show prospective employees how they "walk the talk" after new employees are hired. A variety of sources can be used to recruit employees.

The combined skills of marketing and human resources professionals can provide an impressive picture of the organization to prospective employees. Knowing what information to include in a classified advertisement, combined with creative presentation of the information, can set apart an organization from its competitors.

Written and Internet Advertisements

In addition to traditional newspaper advertisements, some organizations are using Internet sources for recruiting—a source that is especially valued by younger workers who are skilled in the use of computer technology. The job description in each of these media should include information about the specific elements of the job and the special qualities of the organization that would make it a desirable place to work. For example, if the organization has adopted total quality management, which promotes employee involvement, empowerment, and development, advertising this might attract additional applicants. Including descriptive information in promotional advertisements also provides candidates an opportunity to eliminate from consideration the jobs or places that do not match their personal needs.

Job Fairs

Providing clinical or "shadowing" experiences to students, as described in Chapter 5, can be a valuable recruiting tool. A representative of the organization should attend job fairs or career days on campus to provide an additional link to students. Sending the right employees to these events can help recruit the right employees. For example, if the emphasis of a particular career day is on nursing, it is helpful to have a nurse from the organization in attendance to answer specific questions from the students. A positive testimonial from a current employee can send a powerful message to job seekers.

Hiring from Within the Organization

Internal candidates may be the best candidates for jobs in the organization. Although there is value in adding people from outside to provide new perspectives, it has been suggested that only 20 percent of positions should be filled by individuals from outside the organization (Pinsker, 1991, p. 44). Internal candidates are not the appropriate choices for every job, but when there are qualified employees there are advantages to hiring from within the organization, including enhanced employee morale, motivation, and commitment to the organization. Failure to promote from within can lead to frustration on the part of employees, making it difficult for the outside people who join the organization to be effective (Morgan and Smith, 1996, p. 236). Organizations may also lose high-quality employees who look for opportunities elsewhere once they have been passed over in favor of an outsider.

Executive Search Firms

Search firms are often used for recruiting management-level employees. Although this can be an expensive option, it may be the best way to locate applicants who have the leadership skills needed to help an organization in the process of making substantial changes.

Other recruitment activities may be considered based on unique features of an organization or community. To make the best use of dollars allocated to recruiting, organizations benefit from continuously monitoring the effectiveness of the various sources they use and making changes as indicated (Morgan and Smith, 1996, pp. 221–227).

The Interview

Good hiring decisions begin with preparation for the interview. Preparation includes making decisions about the length of the interview, the questions that will be asked, and who will be involved in the interview. Unfortunately, "most job seekers are more prepared for employment interviews than the people who hire them" (Hacker, 1996, p. 93). Interviewers should keep in mind their responsibility of "selling" the prospective employees on the value of the organization.

Behavioral Interview Questions

The goal of behavioral interview questions is to try to determine how a prospective employee would respond to various situations that may occur in the workplace. These questions are based on the premise that past behavior is a good predictor of future performance. The questions are designed to measure a variety of skills as well as the manner in which the candidate performed the skills. Following is a list of behavioral questions that should be asked of the candidate and the corresponding skills they measure:

- *Goal setting:* Give an example of an important goal that you have set in the past and talk about your success in reaching it.
- *Leadership:* Give an example of a time in which you feel you were able to build motivation in your coworkers.
- *Coping:* Describe a time on any job that you've held in which you were faced with problems or stresses that tested your coping skills. What did you do?

- *Organization and planning:* Give an example that demonstrates your ability to organize tasks.
- *Creativity:* Describe the most creative work-related project that you have carried out.
- *Team building:* Give an example of a time when you were part of a team that performed especially well.
- *Initiative:* Give an example of a time when you had to go above and beyond the call of duty in order to get a job done.
- *Communication:* Describe a situation in which your communication skills helped you to market an idea or concept to a customer.
- *Decision making:* Describe a situation in which you had to make an important decision without all available information.
- *Assertiveness:* Give an example of a time when you used facts and reason to persuade another person to take action.
- *Conflict management:* Give an example of a time when you disagreed with your supervisor and describe how the situation was resolved.
- *Flexibility:* Describe a situation that required you to assume responsibilities in addition to your regular workload.

The answers to these questions will provide information about the candidate's values while also providing an opportunity for the interviewers to observe the candidate's verbal communication skills and nonverbal behavior.

Various sources of information about effective interview questions are available for those who would like to expand their current inventory of questions. In the book *Sharkproof*, Mackay (1993) includes a list of twenty complex and revealing interview questions. The late Dr. Kurt Einstein, a behavioral psychologist who was a trainer for both executives and job seekers for many years, compiled the list. Insights by both Mackay and Einstein about what the answers of the candidate reveal are also included. Every question may not be appropriate for every interview, but the list provides some thought-provoking ways to assess the work values of prospective employees. There are many other reputable sources of information on the subject of behavioral interviewing; this particular one is mentioned because it is widely available to job-seekers. As prospective employees become more knowledgeable about interviewing strategies, it becomes even more essential for interviewers to continue to actively prepare for interviews.

Identifying Potential Problem Behavior

Before deciding which interview questions to ask, it is helpful to have an idea of the type of answers that are appropriate or desired. Various books and articles have been written to explain interview questions and provide insights into the meaning of various responses, especially those responses that may indicate potential problems. The ability to identify these "red flags" can help the employer avoid making poor hiring decisions.

The following questions are designed to provide information about a candidate's interaction with coworkers:

- *Ask candidates to describe the best and the worst boss they ever had.* If people spend ten minutes talking about the worst situation and two minutes talking about the positive, it may be an indication that they focus on negative rather than positive situations. Evaluating only the time spent on an answer without considering the ideas expressed may not provide the most accurate picture of the candidates, however. The choice of adjectives or other terminology may also provide clues about how the candidates communicate with coworkers or supervisors.

- *Ask candidates to describe a situation in which they experienced failure and what was learned from it.* The answers to these questions provide insight into some of the candidates' behavioral traits. Do they blame others for their own failure, or do they

take responsibility for the lessons learned from the experience? The answers may reveal information about their attitudes in general and also provide clues about how individuals
accept responsibility for their actions.

- *Ask candidates how they solve problems at work.* Were problems
  solved by working together with others, or do candidates have
  a "straighten them out" attitude toward previous coworkers?
  (adapted from DeBecker, 1997, pp. 191–195)

While interviewers would prefer not to dwell on negative scenarios or appear to be "interrogating" the candidate, a few questions like the ones above may provide some valuable insights into
past behavior. Answers to this type of difficult question may reveal
whether the candidate handles difficult situations in a responsible
manner or uses inappropriate interventions.

Questions the Best Candidates Ask

Job candidates are encouraged to ask questions during an interview
as part of the process of determining whether the organization is a
good match for their skills. Some candidates may limit their questions to asking for clarification about issues that have already been
discussed during the interview. The best candidates are likely to ask
questions that will require thought and preparation on the part of
the interviewer. Questions that the best candidates will ask may
include the following:

- What does the company do to support the community?
- How are individuals here made to feel valued and respected?
- How financially stable is the company?
- What resources will I have to do the job?
- How does the company support good customer service? (Still,
  1997, pp. 190–191)

Interview Teams

Some organizations choose a team or panel approach in interviewing candidates for management-level positions, allowing several employees to be involved in the interview process. Using a team approach for other positions provides some of the same benefits. An advantage of this approach is that it allows several interviewers to hear responses from the candidate at the same time. It also allows interviewers to observe the interaction between the candidate and other interviewers (Still, 1997, p. 141).

The following list includes some recommendations to help ensure that the team interview is structured to provide the information needed to make good hiring decisions.

- *Coordinate the interview.* Make sure that each person involved in the interview knows the specific questions he or she is assigned to ask.
- *Avoid overscheduling.* Scheduling too many interviews in one day may leave the interviewers exhausted, resulting in the interviewers not really listening to one or more of the candidates.
- *Determine a setting that will make the candidate feel comfortable.* People who are more comfortable are more likely to be receptive to the variety of questions that will be included in the interview.
- *Decide how long the interview will last.* Just as agendas are important for keeping meetings on track, an agenda or plan for an interview will also keep it on schedule. It is important to maintain control over the interview and avoid allowing a talkative candidate to keep the interviewers from getting the information they need.
- *Review résumés and cover letters before the interview.* Preferably, these documents are reviewed just before the interview to avoid repeating information when there are multiple interviewers (Hacker, 1996, pp. 98–102).

An important step in this approach to interviewing is to remind the participating employees about illegal questions and plan in advance the specific questions that will be part of the interview.

Following the formal interview, a member of the interview team can give the candidate a tour of the work area and observe the questions and behavior of the candidate in the actual work environment. If this approach is used, it is essential for employees to keep in mind that the interview is still in progress, and it is important to avoid asking inappropriate questions in this less formal environment.

Scoring Grids

A tool that is familiar to quality management professionals is a scoring grid or matrix, which can be used to add an element of objectivity to the interview process. The interview team identifies criteria that are important to consider for a specific position. Job criteria are listed in a column at the top of a page. A column at the left side of the page includes the names of the job candidates. Each member of the interview team independently ranks the individual candidates on a scale of one to five, with one being the low score.

Examples of criteria that might be included in this type of matrix are

- Experience working with teams
- Knowledge of a systematic process improvement model
- Problem-solving skills
- Enthusiasm for teamwork

Whether an interview team uses a formal scoring grid or a less structured list of qualifications, participants should not discuss their impressions or comments until all members of the team have had a chance to form their own impressions. Ideally, the interview team consists of three to five people who are all knowledgeable about the job requirements. The members of the team meet after all of the interviews are completed and reach consensus on which candidate is best for the job (Morgan and Smith, 1996, pp. 381–383).

Follow-up

An essential follow-up to the interview is to check the candidate's references. For some employers, this is automatic; others, however, fail to check references because they believe former employers will say only positive things about the prospective employee. However, the use of open-ended questions to verify dates and other information on the candidate's application or résumé can open the door for the individual to confirm responsibilities the person had in the previous position (DeBecker, 1997, pp. 190–191).

Increasing concerns about violence in the workplace underscore the value of checking references. Organizations may have conservative policies about sharing information in reference checks; however, thorough reference checks may occasionally help to identify potential problems.

Another essential follow-up activity involves communication with all applicants. Every candidate is a customer, if only for a limited time, and should be treated with respect. Impressions that are made during the recruiting and interview process create the overall impression of the organization for the candidate. A negative experience can leave someone with a lasting negative image of the entire organization. Ideally, every candidate leaves the interview experience with the impression that people in the organization acted in a professional and courteous manner. This can be accomplished by making the following steps part of the routine follow-up to the interview:

- Acknowledge all inquiries or applications, if possible.
- Organize the interview process in a way that makes the best use of the applicant's time, designating one person in the organization to coordinate the process.
- Inform all candidates of the anticipated time frames for all aspects of the interview process.

- Inform all candidates once a hiring decision has been made (Morgan and Smith, 1996, pp. 211–212).

Promotion of Organizational Values

The culture of an organization has been described as "the values and beliefs that the company enforces" (Ellig, 1998, p. 175). The culture relies on more than creating mission, vision, or values statements and displaying copies in a prominent location. Dr. Brian Wong states that health care has "created a curious juxtaposition of beautiful buildings and hostile environments" (Mycek, 1998, p. 30). These hostile environments can have a negative influence on external customers and at the same time alienate employees.

If the organization is to retain the best workers after hiring them, it needs to have a plan for continuing to promote the behavior it has identified as critical to its success. Statements that define the values or culture of the organization should be incorporated into every job description. Behavioral objectives for employees can be incorporated into job-specific competencies for every employee. Sharing this information with prospective employees helps them to understand the values of the organization in a tangible way.

Case Studies

Rosenbluth Travel

Rosenbluth Travel has been named one of the top ten in *Fortune* magazine's "100 Best Companies to Work for in America." The owner of the company, Hal Rosenbluth, describes the unique aspects of his company in the book *The Customer Comes Second* (Rosenbluth and Peters, 1992). As mentioned in Chapter 5, the first priority for Rosenbluth Travel in recruiting employees is to find people who are "nice." Rosenbluth believes that a person's job history too often carries more weight during an interview than the person's values. The selection process in his company places more emphasis on kindness, compassion, and unselfishness than on technical skills or formal education. The philosophy is that nice people do better work.

Rosenbluth Travel interviews approximately eight to ten people for a job before making a final selection. The interview process has some unique features that assist efforts to find out what a candidate's true personality is. Some people are very skilled in the art of interviewing well and actual personality traits will not show up unless the candidate participates in some nontraditional activities. For example, the company often places candidates in scenarios that have nothing to do with the company or the job itself. One test that is sometimes used is a driving test. Observing the behavior of someone who is driving may reveal clues about personality traits that may be carried over into the workplace. Another test involves the candidate in a sporting event. The person who values teamwork and plays unselfishly is likely to be viewed as a positive addition to the company.

Candidates for top leadership positions in the company are evaluated by a corporate psychologist and a team of employees in leadership positions. The psychologist's assessment analyzes strengths and weaknesses, values, and personality traits of the candidate (Rosenbluth and Peters, 1992, pp. 51–59).

Many organizations do not use the types of hiring practices described in this case study because of time or financial constraints. The culture of the organization and the community also help determine appropriate practices. Leaders in organizations benefit from benchmarking against a variety of other companies to find ways to improve hiring practices. Individual organizations must decide how to make the best use of their limited resources in the recruiting, interviewing, and hiring processes.

McMurry Publishing

At McMurry Publishing,* CEO Preston McMurry believes that "of all the things we do in business, the single most important

---

*This case study is based on an interview with Preston McMurry, CEO, McMurry Publishing, in Phoenix in December 1998.

thing is to hire people. Because it is the people who produce the product. It's awfully obvious, but it's not often implemented." Nobody gets a job at McMurry until they complete a five-step process.

The first step in the process is to give the prospective employee a copy of a performance evaluation form prior to the first interview. Says Preston, "We've had people take one look at that and leave." The second step is the first interview, which includes an "intimate discussion about values—theirs and ours."

As the third step, final candidates are interviewed by Preston. "I don't make the ultimate decision, but I want to make sure we hire for attitude first." In the fourth step, everyone who interviewed the candidate gets together as a group to discuss how that person would fit in, what his or her strengths and weaknesses are, and what it as a company would need to provide for their orientation.

The fifth step is an orientation plan. When a decision to hire is made, the new employee's sponsor (supervisor) writes a thirty-, sixty-, and ninety-day orientation plan of how he or she hopes to guarantee this person's success: listing the new employee's strengths, what weaknesses need work, and what he or she needs to learn.

"It's time-consuming, but we're not only talking about quality product. This is the single most significant company cost," says Preston.

References

DeBecker, G. *The Gift of Fear*. New York: Dell, 1997.

Ellig, B. R. "Employment and Employability: Foundation of the New Social Contract." *Human Resources Management*, summer 1998, 37(2).

Hacker, C. A. *The Costs of Bad Hiring Decisions and How to Avoid Them*. Delray Beach, Fla: St. Lucie Press, 1996.

Jamieson, D., and O'Mara, J. *Managing Workforce 2000: Gaining the Diversity Advantage*. San Francisco: Jossey-Bass, 1991.

Mackay, H. B. *Sharkproof*. New York: Harper Business, 1993.

Micco, L. "Gallup Study Links Worker Beliefs, Increased Productivity." *HR-News*, Society for Human Resources Management, Sept. 1998.

Morgan, R. B., and Smith, J. E. *Staffing the New Workplace: Selecting and Promoting for Quality Improvement*. Milwaukee: ASQC Quality Press, 1996.

Mycek, S. "Leadership for a Healthy 21st Century." *Healthcare Forum Journal*, July/Aug. 1998.

Pinsker, R. J. *Hiring Winners*. New York: AMACOM, 1991.

Rosenbluth, H. F., and Peters, D. M. *The Customer Comes Second*. New York: Quill William Morrow, 1992.

Still, D. J. *High Impact Hiring: How to Interview and Select Outstanding Employees*. Dana Point, Calif.: Management Development Systems, 1997.

Chapter Seven

Training and Performance Development

Regulatory agencies define mandatory elements of training for health care organizations; for example, the Occupational Safety and Health Administration (OSHA) requirement to train employees who will have contact with hazardous chemicals or blood and body fluids. Beyond the required training, the philosophy of an organization's leaders determines whether the focus of training is to be on maintaining an acceptable level of competence or promoting excellent performance.

The approach to training and development seems to be haphazard in some health care organizations. Training activities may be implemented based on reaction to a pressing issue that has surfaced or as a result of successful training programs observed in other organizations. The most effective training and development approaches follow one of Covey's (1989) recommendations in his well-known book *Seven Habits of Highly Effective People*. Decisions about training and development ideally "begin with the end in mind." Training activities that are designed to contribute to meeting the organization's strategic goals and that are measured both qualitatively and quantitatively are more likely to contribute to the organization's long-term success. This seems to be a more thoughtful approach than reaction to immediate crises or competitive situations.

Levels of Training and Development

The health care industry is largely composed of skilled and professional workers who are certified, registered, licensed, or otherwise credentialed in their particular areas of expertise. Organizations may choose to offer on-site continuing education programs or designate funds for training in their recruiting and retention strategies. Various health care licensing organizations require a designated number of continuing education hours for professionals to maintain their status. Assisting employees' efforts to maintain their professional education requirements may help meet requirements of regulatory agencies; it may also be used as a retention tool. Many professionals need to participate in continuing education regardless of their employers' involvement. Individuals may be more likely to select an employer who supports continuing education through tuition reimbursement plans, flexible scheduling, financial support for development activities, or on-site development opportunities.

The American Society for Training and Development reports that 15,000 U.S. employers (0.5% of all employers) offer 90 percent of the training that is offered each year in the workplace. The average American company spends less than 1 percent of its payroll on training (McDonald, 1996, p. 32). Many companies offer no formal training, relying instead on an informal on-the-job learning approach. This informal training, which introduces people to the culture and social networks within the organization, relies on experienced employees to informally share information about how the work gets done. At first glance, an informal approach may appear to be less expensive. However, a 1990 study reported that informal training costs ranged from $90 to $180 billion a year for employers, while formal training cost approximately $30 billion (Ford, 1997, p. 129). In the absence of a structured approach to orientation, new employees are more likely to make mistakes that lead to rework. When performance expectations are not clear, misunderstandings and extended learning time are likely to occur. A structured, formal approach to orientation helps employees learn their role in a supportive environment.

Companies that have made a commitment to training efforts believe they have invested in more than a perk or an employment trend. In addition to required training programs, they support continuing education that helps employees develop personal effectiveness both inside and outside the workplace. They also invest in technology to provide technical and college courses on-site. They are developing skills to better prepare employees for the future through work-based education (Atkinson, 1994, p. 60).

Ideally, the strategic goals of an organization should help to define the financial resources that need to be devoted to training. An equally important consideration is the desired end result of training. The goal of training may be any one or a combination of the following:

- A recruitment and retention tool
- A way to help ensure a level of competence or expertise
- A tool to improve the quality of employees' lives, thereby improving work performance

Whether training is coordinated by one designated department or by individual departments, it needs to be designed to contribute to strategic goals. If training efforts are intended to contribute to organizational goals, they ideally should flow from the initial interview process and be continued throughout the employment experience of employees.

Justifying Training Programs

Justification for training programs is a difficult yet necessary fact of life in health care and other industries. Sharing a philosophical belief that training or educating employees will pay dividends in recruitment, retention, customer service, or cost savings is one of the first steps to justifying the costs of training. However, if the organization does not have a clear understanding of the costs associated with failing to adequately train employees, they may opt to eliminate many training and/or development programs.

When faced with limited resources, health care organizations may offer required training to their employees whereas development activities may be reduced or eliminated. Benchmarking with health care and other organizations possessing strong commitments to training and development can provide some data to help justify both expenses. References to specific organizations and global trends can help trainers present a more persuasive case for increased training and development activities.

Scott Parry, chairman and founder of Training House, Inc., was recently inducted into the Human Resources Development Hall of Fame for his expertise in justifying training costs. Parry states, "Training isn't just a soft and squishy thing. It can be engineered to produce very specific results" (Kiser, 1999, p. 80). Testimonials of leaders in the industry can be helpful, but these anecdotal endorsements of training cannot be used alone in efforts to justify costs of training. Administrators must be cost conscious, so the benefits must also be presented in financial terms. Programs that focus on "soft skills" or "attitudes" are the most difficult to measure quantitatively.

Many business leaders believe that people are their company's most important asset. As previously noted, health care often falls behind other businesses in terms of financially investing in this particular asset. According to consultant Tom McDonald (1996, p. 32), the minds and hearts of people drive the growth strategy of an organization. Neglecting the development of people is "tantamount to neglecting your business."

Defining the Need

Some specific training needs are determined by the nature of the services provided in the organization. Agencies that regulate practice standards provide guidelines for minimum competency requirements. Beyond meeting these standards, the defined need for training within an organization changes over time, depending on its day-to-day priorities and long-term strategic goals.

Marshall Kreuter, President of Health 2000, previously worked for the Centers for Disease Control to develop program guidelines for agencies offering community health programs. Kreuter suggests a simplified strategy for determining the health needs of a community by asking the following questions:

1. What is the problem?
2. Who has it?
3. Why do they have it?
4. What can we do about it?

This same simplified formula could be applied to defining the training needs of the community that exists within a health care organization. Answering these core questions helps define whether the issue or problem can be successfully resolved with training alone or with training in conjunction with other interventions.

1. *What is the problem?* Conversely, what are the potential problems if no training takes place? Can training alone solve the problem?

2. *Who has it?* Is there new information or a goal that all employees need to know about, or is there information that affects only employees in a designated area?

3. *Why do they have it?* Do the employees affected by the problem need training? Do they have access to all of the tools and knowledge needed to work efficiently?

4. *What can we do about it?* Is training within the financial and personnel resources of the organization? Does providing training in this particular area enhance the organization's goals? What are the consequences of providing no training?

Finally, the most important question is related to the idea of beginning with the end in mind. A training program is usually not the desired end result; the formal training program is just one of the steps leading to the end result. Alan Todd, CEO of KnowledgeSoft, believes the focus of training needs to shift from tabulating the number of people who participated in training to ensuring that a company has the "right people in the right place with the right knowledge to execute your business plan" (Stamps, 1999, p. 45).

Internal Versus External Trainers

Once a decision has been made to provide training in a specific content area, the decisions about how to offer the training need to be made. An important consideration is weighing the benefits of internal versus external trainers or facilitators. Trainers from outside the organization may be consultants whose expertise is in leading groups or providing presentations focused on a particular topic. These experts may be able to provide information based on current research and trends in the field. An advantage of hiring an external consultant is the objective approach the consultant can provide the organization. A perception often exists that someone from outside the organization has more expertise than trainers within the organization. However, a popular whimsical definition among trainers is that an expert is "a person from out of town who carries a briefcase." The disadvantage of contracting the services of an external trainer is the added costs associated with the consultant's presentation and travel fees. Financial constraints may also prevent an external consultant's involvement in follow-up activities beyond the initial assessment and training stages.

One of the reasons organizations may opt to use in-house trainers is to reduce expenses. Another advantage of in-house trainers is their ability to adapt the content or methods of presentations as needed over a period of time. Familiarity with the organization's goals and social culture is also a valuable tool for trainers who consistently provide this service. These trainers work within the culture on a day-to-day basis.

Whether an organization opts for internal or external sources to provide training, the focus needs to remain on providing the kinds of training and development activities that will keep employees working consistently toward organizational goals.

Defining Behavioral Expectations of Employees

When training is aligned with organizational goals, one of the desired outcomes is that employees understand not only job responsibilities but also behavioral expectations.

Once the expectations of employees are defined within the context of the organization's strategic goals, the information needs to be communicated consistently to employees in a variety of stages, including the initial interview, the orientation program, performance appraisal discussions, and training and development programs.

The Initial Interview

The initial employment interview helps clarify the skills of job applicants. It also provides an opportunity for the employer to begin the process of defining expectations. An overview of the strategic goals emphasizes the commitment of the organization to each individual's role in contributing to these goals. The Disney organization is well known for its method of clarifying expectations during the initial interview process. Explanations of dress code and expected behavior toward other employees and customers are explained at this time. If prospective employees do not feel that they will be able to comply with the expectations, they have the option of leaving at that time with no adverse consequences.

The Orientation Program

After the employee has been hired, the next step is the formal orientation process. Many health care organizations provide an initial one-day or two-day orientation program for all new employees. Usually, the format is a classroom setting in which information is provided to new employees about the history, mission, and goals of the organization. Other topics may include safety information and details about programs unique to the organization. It is also the setting where priorities such as customer service or continuous quality improvement are described. New employee orientation is a valuable marketing tool for the organization. It is an opportunity to highlight successes and ensure that new employees leave at the end of the day feeling confident, excited, and committed to a high-quality organization. Reviewing expectations during this initial orientation helps new employees understand how their actions contribute to the organization's ability to maintain its quality standards.

This initial orientation is essential not only for providing information, but also for introducing individuals to other new employees and beginning to define the social structure of the organization. Special perks, such as a complimentary lunch or a small gift are often provided at this time to give new employees a warm welcome to the organization. The process of welcoming new employees does not have to end with the general orientation. While it may be necessary to get the job-specific orientation started immediately following the general orientation, efforts to continue the socialization process can be incorporated into the next phase of orientation.

A letter to the editor of a nursing journal once described an orientation process for a public school teacher. The writer explained that her daughter had recently started her first job as a teacher. When she arrived at the school for the required teachers' meetings, she found that her classroom had been decorated and her coworkers had planned a welcome reception. The writer, who had been a nurse for many years, suggested that we in health care could learn a lesson from this experience. The message is that we should put more effort into the way we welcome new employees.

Preceptor or Mentor Programs

Nursing departments often use a preceptor or mentor approach to job-specific orientation. Disciplines other than nursing benefit from expanding their orientation program to include this approach.

An important role of preceptors is to model the expected behaviors in conjunction with other aspects of their jobs. Preceptors can be rewarded for the extra work associated with that role in a variety of ways, from financial incentives to additional time off work. Recognition of the extra work required also requires adjusting the preceptor's usual workload accordingly; otherwise, the preceptor is not able to devote the time and attention needed to guide the new employee through the orientation process. The financial implications of adjusting workloads for preceptors need to be considered during the budgeting process in order for the process to work efficiently.

A preceptor approach also benefits the new employee by providing a consistent resource person during the orientation process. New employees may be hesitant to ask too many questions, fearing that their coworkers will think they are not doing a good job. Preceptors are trained to anticipate the questions and fears of new employees.

The goal of becoming a preceptor can be incorporated into the professional development plans for employees in both clinical and nonclinical departments. If preceptors are to be successful, expectations of the preceptor role must be clearly communicated, preferably through a formal classroom training process. Preceptor workshops are offered by various health care organizations. If an organization does not have the resources in-house to offer this type of training program, employees may be able to attend a program at an off-site location for a nominal fee. Examples of general topics that are often incorporated into the formal training program include the following:

- Planning and organizing the orientation
- Providing constructive feedback to the orientee and staff
- Problem-solving strategies
- Continuously evaluating the orientation process

Preceptor training reinforces the need for ongoing feedback about an employee's performance. New employees also evaluate the preceptor program at various stages throughout the orientation process. The data collected can provide useful information for maintaining and improving this approach to orientation.

Performance Appraisals

The place where most employees expect to see an evaluation of skills and behavior is in the performance appraisal form. Many health care organizations choose to implement an annual performance review. Along with evaluating whether specific duties were or were not accomplished, the performance appraisal should be a working document outlining personal goals for improvement. To increase the likelihood of success the employee and the supervisor should mutually agree on the goals.

Once the underlying structure is in place to help define, reinforce, and evaluate specific expectations of employees, methods of training and empowering employees to reach goals must be implemented. A poorly designed system will eventually defeat even the best worker (Just, Towner-Larsen, and Wittman, 1998).

Empowering Employees

A key aspect of empowerment is keeping employees aware of some basic guidelines for decision making. Problems with empowerment can arise when it is viewed as a separate entity from the goals of the company. In recent years, some businesses have focused on reengineering to redefine the way they do business. Efforts to reengineer may encourage employees to throw away old ideas and start over with new, creative ones. Companies that successfully empower employees realize that some structure is necessary for the concept of empowerment to be effective. Employees need access to information that will help guide their decisions. Radical change is appropriate and beneficial if employees understand how to make changes within the framework of the company's business objectives. Companies that promote empowerment want their employees to "use their heads, to solve problems, to make smart decisions" (Case, 1998, pp. 67–68).

The health care industry depends on individuals to provide high-quality patient care by carefully following policies and procedures. The idea of being a risk taker is intimidating to some health care workers because of the nature of the work they do. Hospitals designate individuals to function as risk managers. The word *risk* is closely associated with a negative outcome. The focus on safety becomes so ingrained that risk taking in any context creates an uncomfortable feeling. Empowering health care workers to be creative or flexible requires thoughtful definition of the structures that support independent decision making.

For example, many quality improvement theories rely on the use of teams to analyze processes and design improvements. Employees need access to data about how those processes work, along with guidelines defining the financial constraints for changing a particular process. Employees need to understand how their financial recommendations will affect the overall business plan of the organization. Defining how much money a team will be able to access can make the difference between the team's success or failure.

Empowerment also requires that employees understand their accountability for the outcome of their participation in the decision-making process (Case, 1998, p. 68). Unfortunately, the concept of accountability often has a negative connotation. The word *accountability* is often synonymous with the word *blame*. The well-known book *The Oz Principle* explains in detail how to promote accountability in individuals to improve organizations. The authors describe at length how to develop an attitude of accountability that focuses on "current and future efforts, rather than reactive and historical explanations" (Connors, Smith, and Hickman, 1994, p. 65). This is another example of common terminology that people may think is self-explanatory; in reality the term can have entirely different meanings to different people.

Defining Terminology

In a book that defines the appropriate use of employee awards programs, Leverence (1997, p. 120) notes that "rules have a tendency to be written as reactions to flaws in the system, rather than as proactive guidelines that anticipate and correct the flaws."

While this observation specifically refers to rules about awards, it is often true of policies as well. Terminology used in policies may be based on previous problems or rule infractions.

A well-known principle of adult learning recognizes the value of presenting information in a variety of ways to increase the likelihood that learning takes place. Preceptors in organizations are encouraged to get as many of the senses involved as possible in learning experiences for new employees. Reading a policy or procedure does not promote learning as effectively as reading, hearing an explanation, and practicing the skill. Even when there is recognition of this concept in the orientation process, many important policies are left for the employee to read in a manual or an employee handbook.

Introducing case studies into department or unit meetings can increase understanding of terms and ideas. Discussion of hypothetical cases allows employees a safe forum in which to ask questions and clarify organizational rules or policies. This requires some advance planning on the part of the person leading the meeting or the involvement of a trainer or facilitator. The benefit is being able to openly define the organization's definition of concepts such as *empowerment* or *accountability*.

Performance Development

Performance development advances training beyond the realm of building work skills. One goal is to enable employees to contribute to achieving the organization's goals by understanding how their day-to-day work contributes to those goals. Another desired result of performance development is to help employees discover ways to contribute to the organization's success while contributing to their own personal development.

Performance appraisals often focus on a review of behavior and accomplishments that have occurred over a previous period, usually one year. A section of the appraisal may be devoted to personal development. Employees who understand how to incorporate personal goals into growth within the organization are more likely to be focused on their work.

Training continues to be a component of development; however, it is not an adequate replacement for performance development. "Companies need to quit thinking in terms of training, and start thinking about knowledge creation and knowledge transfer as distinct and important business processes. The question is not, How do we deliver training to x number of people? It is, How do you make sure you have the right people in the right place with the right knowledge to execute your business plan?" (Stamps, 1999, p. 45)

Dana Gaines Robinson and James C. Robinson have created a systematic approach that can help organizations make the shift from traditional training to performance development. Table 7.1 provides a visual overview of the differences between the two approaches.

The output produced by a performance-focused function is an improved process and/or improved human performance in support of business goals.

The Robinsons compare the process of making the transition from traditional training to performance development with changing a tire on a moving vehicle. Some regulations mandate training that must be completed in health care organizations, and state health departments, the Joint Commission, and OSHA define specific training requirements for health care employees. Deciding on the level of training beyond the essentials requires continuous evaluation of the goals of the organization.

The concept of employee development is sometimes approached by organizations as an all-or-nothing proposition—training programs required to maintain competence are at one end of the spectrum, while additional training and development programs that are costly

**Table 7.1. Traditional Versus Performance Approach
to Training and Development.**

Traditional Approach	Performance Approach
Focuses on what people need to learn; training is the end	Focuses on what people need to do; training is a means to an end
Event-oriented	Process-oriented
Reactive	Proactive and reactive
Biased toward a solution	Bias-free toward solutions
Relies on one solution (learning)	Relies on multiple solutions
Can work independently of client partnerships	Must be partnered to a client
Defines front-end assessment as optional; rarely identifies work environment barriers to desired performance	Defines front-end assessment as mandatory; identifies work environment barriers to skill transfer
Typically restricts evaluation of learning to Level I (reaction) and Level II (learning)	Evaluates at all levels, including Level III (performance) and Level IV (operational change)

Reprinted with permission of Partners in Change, Inc. Copyright © 1995, 1998, Partners in Change, Inc.

and difficult to quantify are at the opposite end of the spectrum. In reality, many opportunities exist somewhere in the middle of these two extremes. Benchmarking with other organizations, identifying employment trends in the community, and surveying employees for suggestions about training are all activities that can help organizations define where they need to be on the training continuum.

Expanding the Boundaries of Training

Many university-based distance education programs bring degree programs from college campuses to work settings. Distance learning programs transmit courses live from college campuses to a variety of sites throughout the university's home state. Hospitals as well as other businesses may choose to purchase equipment needed to provide distance learning options to employees and the community. In some cases, employees can actually complete requirements for a degree through courses offered at the workplace. The cost to the organization is minimal once the initial investment in equipment has been made. Distance learning programs were designed for adult learners who want to pursue advanced degrees, but do not have the ability to travel to a college campus. These classes provide direct interaction between the students and the instructor and between students at various sites. Many universities offer courses and degree programs on the Internet, and the number of courses is increasing. These courses are popular with people who are comfortable with the technology and need flexibility to continue their education.

Hospitals may look to other health care organizations, local businesses, or colleges in the community to share training resources. Managing change, communicating effectively, and providing high-quality customer service are examples of topics that can be provided to employees from a variety of organizations. Sharing training resources may also provide a valuable method of benchmarking with other organizations to discover creative new ways of changing processes.

Measuring Employee Satisfaction

Companies that are recognized as good places to work promote communication to determine employee as well as customer satisfaction. Employee surveys can provide valuable information to employers when a few important guidelines are followed. A good survey includes information about many of the topics previously addressed in these pages:

- Vision, values, and mission of the organization
- Communication between departments as well as between employees and their supervisors
- Reward and recognition programs
- Training and personal development opportunities
- Overall job satisfaction (Penson, 1998, p. 20)

The entire process of giving a survey needs to be carefully planned before the survey is distributed. Following some of the basic principles of a quality improvement approach, establish a timeline that clearly defines steps, dates, and responsibilities of the various people involved in the process. Employees are not likely to participate in a survey if they are not convinced that follow-up of some kind will occur. One of the fears of organizational leaders is that employees will expect all of their suggestions to be implemented. Limiting the number of open-ended questions can help decrease expectations of changes the organization is not able to implement.

The data collected from employee surveys can be used to make changes that will improve both recruitment and retention activities. Communicating the results and any changes that are made based on the information received is critical to the success of future surveys.

Training and development activities are critical to the success of people and the organizations they support. Whether the approach that is used is developed by the individual organization or purchased from a consultant or company, it should be clearly communicated at every step and aligned with the overall direction of the organization.

Case Study: People-Centered Teams Healing the Workplace at St. Charles Medical Center

As a result of a restructuring effort that began in 1992, St. Charles Medical Center in Bend, Oregon, implemented the People-Centered Teams: Healing the Workplace program (Vallerga and Carmichael, 1997). St. Charles supports the philosophy that the healing environment is enhanced by combining both the science and the art of patient care. Patients come to hospitals assuming a level of technical competence, but true healing takes place as a result of the quality of relationships they find there. The key product the organization offers to patients is who its caregivers are and how they work together. The goals for participants of People-Centered Teams training are to:

- Develop trust and internal resourcefulness
- Revitalize enthusiasm and morale
- Communicate effectively
- More fully contribute to their work and the people they serve

People-Centered Teams training is intended for employees at all levels of the organization. The People-Centered Teams seminar is two and one-half days long and usually includes about thirty-five to forty people. Participants explore how their own personal belief systems determine the level of satisfaction they experience and how that influences the degree to which the organization satisfies its customers. Objectives for the workshop include:

- Identifying belief systems and behavior that can support them in getting more of what they want
- Learning to create healthier relationships through improved personal awareness, listening, and differentiated communication
- Exploring how broadening their personal comfort zone can increase individual flexibility and internal resourcefulness
- Understanding group development and how groups come together to form synergistic, interdependent teams
- Discovering ways to more fully contribute their unique talents, skills, and experience to the work they do and the people they serve
- Developing a deeper appreciation of how diversity serves to make organizations stronger
- Understanding the stages of change and how to support themselves and others in times of transition
- Learning how the "victim triangle" undermines personal and organizational growth and how to dismantle it
- Exploring how their attitudes, assumptions, and intentions determine the outcomes they obtain
- Developing a personal vision statement to guide them into the future

In-house facilitators and peer coaches were trained to implement the program. Facilitators coordinate and deliver on-site training seminars and help teams by providing training on such topics as communication and group process.

The peer coaches serve as role models, coach coworkers on the concepts taught in the seminar, and help them resolve difficult issues. The peer coaches can provide the difference between a one-time training session and a true cultural shift within the organization.

Results experienced by St. Charles after implementing this program include:

- Improvement in patient satisfaction surveys
- A 36 percent decrease in patient accidents
- A 33 percent decrease in employee accidents
- Improvement in employee satisfaction surveys, even in the midst of change
- Cost savings in hours per adjusted patient discharge
- The highest Joint Commission survey score ever

In addition to these results, there are positive anecdotal outcomes. One manager reported spending only 3 percent of his time managing conflict, versus 32 percent prior to the implementation of the program. Comments in employee surveys report the employees' increased satisfaction with their ability to resolve conflicts and complaints. They believe they are more willing to address concerns because of the skills they acquired in the training sessions. Prior to the training, they would not have had the confidence to address uncomfortable issues. Other comments from employees include:

- People greet one another in the hallway and mean it.
- There is more willingness to work together.
- People seem to genuinely enjoy their work.
- There has been a shift in focus from perfection to excellence.

St. Charles Medical Center has created a plan for ongoing implementation of this process. In addition to providing training to facilitators and peer counselors, the organization depends on its "Healing Healthcare" management team to oversee implementation of the process in coordination with the long-term organizational vision. The training sessions are not mandatory. Employees are generally willing to attend, based on positive feedback from others who have attended the sessions.

References

Atkinson, M. "Build Learning into Work." *HR Magazine*, Sept. 1994, 39(9).

Case, J. *The Open Book Experience: Lessons from Over 100 Companies Who Successfully Transformed Themselves*. Reading, Mass.: Addison Wesley, 1998.

Connors, R., Smith, T., and Hickman, C. *The Oz Principle—Getting Results Through Individual and Organizational Accountability*. Paramus, N.J.: Prentice Hall, 1994.

Covey, S. R. *The Seven Habits of Highly Effective People*. New York: Simon & Schuster, 1989.

Ford, K. *Improving Training Effectiveness in Work Organizations*. Mahwah, N.J.: Erlbaum, 1997.

Just, J., Towner-Larsen, B., and Wittman, N. "Performance Consulting: Notes from the Field." Conference presentation, "Healthcare Management, Staff Development, and Education: Strategies for Success," Columbus, Ohio, Oct. 7, 1998.

Kiser, K. "Move Over, Nerds." *Training*, Jan. 1999, 36(1).

Leverence, J. *And the Winner Is—Using Awards Programs to Promote Your Company and Encourage Your Employees*. Santa Monica: Merritt Publishing, 1997.

McDonald, T. "The Learning Tree." *Successful Meetings*, Nov. 1, 1996, 45(12).

Penson, P. G. "Employee Surveys Are Worth Plenty if Done Right." *Sacramento Business Journal*, Sept. 18, 1998, 15(27).

Stamps, D. "Enterprise Training: This Changes Everything." *Training*, Jan. 1999, 36(1).

Vallerga, L., and Carmichael, B. "People-Centered Teams: Healing the Workplace." Conference presentation, American Society for Education and Training annual meeting, Orlando, Fla., May 4, 1997.

Chapter Eight

Structuring Employee Benefits

Underlying structures are required to support the mission, vision, and values of an organization. These structures give employees the ability to go beyond familiarity with the organization's goals by having the resources to act on them. It is not necessary to merge the marketing and human resources departments or rewrite the organizational chart to make this happen. Systematically selecting new or revised practices can improve the interaction of these two essential functions. The use of surveys and focus groups can help employers determine where time and other resources are best used to create positive changes in the organization's culture. If an organization's culture is not positive in supporting employees, it may be perceived as negative. There is no neutral or middle ground (Herman, 1998, p. 1). Evaluating the effectiveness of each change using whatever quality improvement model the organization subscribes to increases the likelihood of success.

Creating and Maintaining the Salary and Benefits Package

Competitive salaries and benefits packages together provide incentives for potential new employees. Surveys suggest that workers want more than just a job. Workers are considering entire packages when making decisions about jobs. They use criteria such as "learning opportunities, family centeredness, social responsibility, flexibility, and spirituality" when deciding where they want to work (Herman, 1998, p. 2).

The 1997 National Study of the Changing Workforce reports that in that year approximately 74 to 84 percent of workers had access to traditional benefits, which included:

- Health insurance coverage
- Pension or retirement plan
- Paid time off, including vacations and holidays
- Paid time off for personal illness (Bond, Galinsky, and Swanberg, 1998)

These benefits may be expected by most workers, simply because they have always been a part of the employment package. This chapter will explore some of the changes that are occurring in traditional benefits, as well as innovative changes in benefits offered by some companies.

Health Benefits

Health insurance coverage is a traditional benefit that is undergoing significant changes. The days of health insurance costs paid entirely by the company have become a distant memory to many people in the workforce. Workers now pay on average 25 percent of health care premiums. Health insurance premiums are expected to continue to increase much faster than inflation. The Congressional Budget Office anticipates that inflation will average 2.8 percent over the next decade and health insurance premiums will rise approximately 5.5 percent in that same period (Battistella and Burchfield, 1998, pp. 24–25).

According to Battistella and Burchfield (p. 26), professors of health care policy, low levels of unemployment and shortages in some occupations add to the difficulty of keeping labor costs from increasing. Employers are shifting increases in health premiums to workers by changing levels of coverage or increasing amounts of copayments. Medical savings accounts will likely become increasingly popular with employers as they try to control rising health care costs. Health care organizations are not exempt from these inevitable changes in the economy. However, they have processes in place to monitor and analyze costs of health coverage for employees. This advantage over other industries could prove helpful in adding innovative benefits to help recruit and retain employees who have skills that could take them to competitors.

Along with the morale issues associated with high turnover, the financial impact can also be significant for organizations, particularly smaller ones. The cost of turnover has been estimated to range between 50 to 150 percent of the annual salary for the position (Kelley, 1998, p. 2). Companies are offering creative incentives in the form of increased benefits in an effort to retain employees. Suggestions include increased vacation time, flextime, job sharing, and wellness time (p. 6).

Even in organizations with limited financial resources, creative benefits may enhance a positive culture that values employees.

Sick Days and Well Days

The need for sick time is an inevitable fact of life. Still, employee wellness programs can affect costs by reducing the number of sick days experienced by employees. Healthier employees also have the ability to be more productive when they are at work. Caregivers sometimes take care of their patients at the expense of their own health.

Caregivers are exposed to elements that cause both physical illness and mental stress. Because of the nature of services provided, the health care industry is an ideal setting for increasing health promotion programs as a benefit for employees. Many industries are exploring health promotion programs as a way to increase employee satisfaction and at the same time create a healthier workforce. This is one area where health care organizations can demonstrate how well they follow their own advice.

Health Promotion

Health promotion is a concept that is gaining increased attention as a way to create a healthier workforce and to reward employees who take steps to prevent illness. Insurers have been getting on the health promotion bandwagon in varying degrees. While the idea of keeping people healthy to reduce health care expenses may seem logical, the numbers to justify the commitment of money to prevention services are sometimes difficult to compile. Health promotion may sound appealing to employers and employees from a theoretical standpoint, but the reality of the costs associated with prevention of illness is sometimes a barrier. Fortunately, research into the health behavior of employees and the corresponding cost saving is increasing.

Employers need to see examples of cost-effectiveness before they will support health promotion activities in addition to the traditional health care coverage provided to employees. The evidence that would help sell the idea of health promotion activities would need to document the following assumptions:

- Individuals with modifiable risk factors for illness cost more than individuals without these risks.
- Improvements in risk factors result in cost reduction.
- Health habits can be changed and maintained over time.
- Benefits of reducing health risks by changing health habits outweigh the costs.

A study conducted from 1990 to 1995 provides data to support the first of these criteria. Health Risk Appraisal (HRA) instruments and health screenings were provided to over 65,000 employees working for six large employers across the country. All six employers were clients of The MEDSTAT Group, located in Ann Arbor, Michigan, and The StayWell Company from St. Paul, Minnesota. Participation in the study was voluntary, with approximately half of the employees electing to participate. The Health

Enhancement Research Organization (HERO) database was used to analyze the relationship between health risks and medical expenditures.

The findings suggested that employees at high risk for health problems had substantially higher expenditures than employees at lower risk in seven of ten modifiable risk categories. The seven factors include the following:

- Depression
- High stress
- High blood glucose
- Extremely over- or underweight
- Tobacco use
- High blood pressure
- Sedentary lifestyle

The average annual medical expenditures for "risk-free" individuals was $1,166. Individuals who smoked, did not exercise, had poor eating habits, had high blood pressure and high cholesterol, and reported being highly stressed averaged annual expenditures of $3,803. Individuals who reported being both depressed and highly stressed were approximately 147 percent more costly than others who did not have those risks (Goetzel and others, 1998, pp. 843–854).

The information presented in this study is significant because of the length of the study and the number of employees involved. The authors of the study conclude that much more research needs to be completed to further explore cost-effectiveness of health promotion activities in the workplace.

Figures 8.1 and 8.2 highlight some of the successes and innovations in contemporary health promotion programs.

A study completed by William M. Mercer Inc. in 1998 determined the extent to which companies were implementing health promotion programs. The report included responses from 259 companies. Of those companies, 55 percent had health management programs,

Figure 8.1. Two Successful Health Promotion Programs.

Coors—In 1990, the Coors wellness program cost approximately $60 per employee. The company saved at least $1.9 million that year in reduced medical costs, decreased sick leave, and increased productivity. The Coors company started the wellness program in 1981, long before most employers were thinking seriously about wellness or health promotion programs.

Reynolds Electrical & Engineering Co. Inc.—The company introduced a wellness program provided by Anthem Health System of Indianapolis. Employees who elected to participate in the program completed a health risk appraisal and received an on-site physical exam. Intervention programs focusing on weight loss, breast health, and stress management were implemented. The results were measured over a two-year period. The program cost was approximately $76 per person, and there was an average decrease of $121 per employee in lifestyle-related claims (Cerrato, 1995, pp. 21–24).

with 63 percent of the companies using some kind of incentive for employees to participate. Incentives improve employee participation in health promotion programs (Ziegler, 1997, p. 27).

Employees are not likely to participate in health promotion programs unless they can be assured of confidentiality. Employers may be advised to use the services of an outside consultant to provide health screenings for this reason. Just as confidentiality is a critical element of any patient care procedure in a health care organization, it must also be guaranteed to employees who participate in health promotion programs.

Flexible Benefits

Flexible benefits, or "cafeteria benefits plans," allow employees to choose and contribute to benefits that best meet their needs. Flexible spending accounts are attractive to some employees who have routine medical expenses that can be paid on a pretax basis. Employees choosing only benefits they know they will use may reduce costs for the employer.

These plans may be attractive to employees but they present some distinct disadvantages for employers. Administering multiple

Figure 8.2. Innovative Health Promotion: Massage Therapy.

Intuit in Mountain View, California, and Cigna Corporation in Philadelphia have introduced massage therapy into their wellness programs as an extension of stress management intervention. Massage breaks were found to be cost-effective, whether partially or totally paid by the company. One study has shown that adults who have two fifteen-minute massages each week showed signs of increased relaxation and increased speed and accuracy of math computations over members of a control group (Woodward, 1998, p. 106).

Memorial Hospital in Chattanooga, Tennessee, implemented massage therapy for employees in an attempt to be as sensitive to employees' needs as to patients' needs. Health care workers, especially nurses, often have difficulty getting away from work areas, so the massages are taken to the workers. There are some liability issues that must be considered before implementing massage therapy as an employee benefit. These include the potential for injury and the concern about potential sexual abuse. These liability issues can be addressed before implementing the practice by thoroughly screening therapists and planning the process carefully (Woodward, 1998, p. 108).

The mere mention of the concept of "massage therapy" or other alternative therapies can create fear among senior management in organizations. Innovative ideas can create so much fear or discomfort that the ideas are abandoned before they are fully investigated. One of the best values of teams in organizations is the ability of several people generating and researching ideas before they are ever proposed as policy changes. Teams help empower employees, who help create an image of a "good place to work." The key is to be able to move out of the comfort zone to explore innovative ideas.

plans can be confusing and time-consuming. Regular communication with employees is essential in order to keep them up to date on changes in the plans as well as their responsibilities. This is especially important as managed care plans are implemented and periodically adjusted. Employees need to be informed of their responsibilities in locating approved providers of care.

Flextime

Many employers are attempting to respond to their employees' need to balance personal and work life by increasing the flexibility of benefits and schedules. Flextime allows workers to adjust the beginning and ending times of their workdays. Flextime is helpful for employees who need to adjust their schedules to school starting times or for elderly parents. Some employers believe that flextime supports employees' efforts to stay focused on their work as a result of having the time they need to take care of personal issues at home. Flextime presents a challenge for health care organizations because of the number of jobs that must have an exact starting time. In some cases, caregivers in a specific work area are willing to work together to create flexible schedules that meet staff needs.

Dependent Care

Dependent care is a term that encompasses not only child care, but also care of elderly relatives. It is estimated that anywhere from 20 to 30 percent of the workforce has responsibility for elder care. The number of missed workdays due to caring for an elderly relative is also increasing. Employers are investigating options for employees with elder care issues to help prevent absenteeism and to reduce stress while the employee is on the job.

Companies tend to be more familiar with child care issues, since they have been dealing with them for a longer period. There are several options for child care benefits:

- *On-site day care*. This option provides parents with the security of having their children close to them while they are at work. Day care centers in hospitals have the added security benefit of immediate emergency care if it should be needed.

- *Child care allowance*. This is a flexible spending account that allows employees to pay day care expenses with pretax dollars and does not have any direct costs for the employer.

- *Day care information*. Referral information about day care or other dependent care options in the area can be helpful to employees, especially new workers who are relocating to the area. Parents may soon be able to look in on their children by logging onto a web site. Some day care centers are setting up cameras that allow parents to check in on their children from work. Employers may need to add this possibility into future benefit considerations for new employees.

- *Flexible scheduling.* In addition to flextime, described previously, job sharing may be an option for some employees who have responsibility for the care of a dependent.

Working Mother magazine regularly reports its assessment of the 100 best companies for working mothers. The results reported in October 1998 considered for the first time whether companies provide managers with training in meeting the personal needs of employees. The reviewers also considered how well these programs are implemented. Texas Instruments is one of the companies that made the list for 1998. The company expects managers to take classes on how to make decisions that consider not only business needs, but also workers' needs. The E.I. duPont de Nemours Company evaluates managers on whether they support employees' personal needs along with their work needs. Some managers in the company are required to take a course on using flexibility as a business tool (Laabs, 1998, p. 56).

Opportunities for Advancement

One of the main reasons people leave organizations is to pursue better opportunities. However, even in small companies, employees may be eligible for better opportunities without leaving the organization. Lands' End in Dodgeville, Wisconsin, allows employees to try out a job in a different area of the company for a short time. If they don't like the new job, they have the option of remaining in their current position (Herman, 1998, p. 2). Just as business is constantly changing, individual employees' needs and priorities will also change over time. The job that was once challenging and exciting may no longer hold the interest of an employee at a later period. Rather than lose a good employee, why not explore whether a better opportunity exists within the walls of the same organization?

Compensation—Not Just Money

Employees expect fair compensation for the work they do. Other forms of compensation include personal recognition, opportunities for professional advancement, and decision-making authority.

There is increasing evidence to support the theory that money is not the primary motivation for either current employees or job seekers. The 1997 National Study of the Changing Workforce reports some of the key components that workers believe are essential to job satisfaction. Although employers may consider wages and traditional fringe benefits to be primary determinants of job satisfaction, employees describe job quality and employer supportiveness as being more important to long-term satisfaction. Job quality includes "autonomy on the job, learning opportunities, meaningfulness of work, opportunities for advancement, and job security." Workplace support includes "flexibility in work arrangements, supervisor support, supportive workplace culture, positive coworker relations, absence of discrimination, respect in the workplace, and equal opportunity for workers of all backgrounds" (Bond, Galinsky, and Swanberg, 1998).

Other research reflects these same priorities for employees. Some of the other qualities workers expect have been presented in previous chapters under various headings. Workers want to make a difference, and they want to spend their working hours in an environment that is caring and supportive of their efforts. How do employers balance these difficult-to-measure traits with traditional wages and benefits?

At times, it seems the needs of employees in a particular organization do not coincide with those described in the research. Responding to the needs of an employee population requires not only an understanding of industry trends but also the unique characteristics of the group. Human resources professionals hear comments that undoubtedly cause them to wonder if the needs of employees in their organization really are different from those expressed elsewhere. Unfortunately, comments like these are too often expressed in health care organizations:

- "I have a friend who works at (competing) hospital, and she makes a lot more money than I do."
- "If you would just pay us what we're worth, we wouldn't have these staffing shortages."

Human resources staff may feel the burden of trying to determine whether workers who make these comments are a vocal minority or if the comments represent the majority of employees. Employees who make such comments may be reacting to a variety of workplace issues. The responsibility for making positive changes does not rest solely with the human resources staff in an organization that has well-thought-out strategic goals and objectives. Managers and supervisors throughout the organization should reward and encourage employees who are working toward the goals and avoid the temptation to spend too much time addressing the employees who do not support change. Behavior that is rewarded will be noticed by other employees. Improving job quality requires much more work than offering new benefits or higher pay scales. It is a matter of changing the organizational structures or culture—a long-term and continuous process.

A small health care provider in the Midwest recently experienced a reduction in funding for its services. The CEO called a staff meeting to announce that while there would be no pay raises, the value of the staff was not represented by the dollars paid. She went on to review some of the benefits, including vacation days, sick days, free meals and parking, and flexible work schedules. She then proceeded to mention each staff member, noting individual contributions to the organization's success and thanking them for their faithful service. Following some discussion of other business matters, the meeting closed with condolences expressed to some of the staff members who had recently experienced deaths in their families. This example illustrates ways to recognize, encourage, and support employees even when difficult compensation issues must be addressed.

Balancing Work and Personal Life

An emerging theme in the workplace as we move into the next millennium is balancing work and personal needs. When HR recruiters go to college campuses, it is not unusual for prospective employees to ask specifically how the organization will help them balance work and personal life. Many prospective employees graduating college will check the web site of an organization. If they don't like what they see within the first couple of minutes, they will exit and look for other opportunities. Companies can provide information on their web sites by using statistics, graphics, and descriptions or a combination of these to tell the story of who they are and what they have to offer employees. Some companies provide a virtual tour of the organization on their web site. This technology makes the concept of a good first impression even more critical.

Companies are offering a variety of innovative benefits to address personal as well as work concerns of employees. Examples of services for employees include prepared meals for employees to take home to their families, on-site dry cleaning and laundry pickup and delivery, film pickup and delivery, and in-house personal shoppers for special-occasion gifts. An article in *Working Woman* magazine highlighting these unique perks, however, questions whether they are designed to "keep people at work longer" (Austin, 1998, p. 21). Employees might actually prefer more time to take care of these errands on their own. The key is to ask employees their opinions before implementing policies that may have the best possible intentions while missing the key ingredients that employees really want. Flexible and unique benefits help with recruitment and retention efforts; they can also influence employee loyalty to the organization. "The more you recognize and address the balancing act that employees go through, the more committed those employees are going to be" (Laabs, 1998, p. 55).

Several studies provide insights into the ways workers would like companies to support the concept of balancing work and personal needs. A few findings from "America at Work," a study conducted by Aon Consulting of Chicago, indicate how priorities of workers are changing:

- In a list of seventeen factors that correlate to employer commitment to the workforce, the top factor is the employer's recognition of the importance of personal and family time. Rounding out the top five were: the organization's overall direction, opportunities for personal growth, ability of employees to influence how things are done, and everyday work satisfaction.

- The percentage of employees who reported job-related burnout increased from 39 percent in 1993 to 53 percent in 1998.

- The average time missed due to stress increased 36 percent since 1995.

- In 1995, 13 percent of survey respondents reported working an average of more than fifty hours per week; in 1998 the number increased to 23 percent (Allerton, 1998, p. 10).

When considering all potential benefits to offer, the most important factor to keep in mind is what the employee wants. This has been measured and reported in a variety of sources, and some generalizations can be made based on research and the experience of similar companies. Individual organizations also have their own specific ways to measure what employees want. All of this information used together can provide employers with information they need in order to remain competitive with other employers.

Aligning Human Resources and Marketing

Integrating specific functions of human resources and marketing does not require placing the two departments together on an organizational chart or changing the reporting relationship of either department. Organizations attempting to align marketing and human resources functions can expect to encounter the same uncomfortable reactions that occur with any kind of organizational change. Organizations may choose at varying times to measure customer satisfaction, implement changes in organizational structure, change the performance evaluation process, or measure employee satisfaction. Aligning marketing and human resources functions may require implementing several of these changes at the same time. Success depends on communication, anticipation of difficulties, and a commitment to a long-term strategy for change.

Cobb, Samuel, and Sexton (1998, pp. 34–40) recommend focused dialogue as a tool to help promote improved communication between people from different areas of an organization. The use of "how" and "what if" questions encourages thoughtful responses to suggested scenarios. The authors cite examples of companies using focussed dialogue prior to implementing changes they believed would be unpopular with employees. Managers asked employees for ideas, asking questions such as:

- What steps would you recommend to solve problems that have been identified?
- How could communication between departments be improved?

In both situations, the managers were pleasantly surprised by the suggestions and the positive reaction of the employees. The focused dialogue technique provides employees the opportunity to express their opinions prior to changes being implemented, which ultimately increases buy-in on their part. These experiences emphasize the importance of avoiding assumptions about how others will react to changes.

People Make the Place

In one large urban hospital, one element of nursing orientation is a session on "how to survive in nursing." This session provides an opportunity for participants to recall when and why they became interested in nursing and why they chose to work in their particular hospital. The reasons for choosing nursing as a career vary, but most often focus on the idea of wanting to "help others" or "make a difference." One of the most compelling reasons for choosing the specific hospital was offered by a woman in her late thirties who waited until her children were in school to pursue her nursing education. She recalled an incident during one of her pregnancies when she became concerned because she had not felt her baby move in what seemed to be a long time. She and her husband were both unemployed, and her next appointment with her doctor was several days away. The harder she tried not to think about it, the more concerned she became that something was wrong with her baby.

The concerned patient called the maternity department and explained her situation to one of the nurses, who advised her to come to the hospital. After she explained the family's financial situation, the nurse instructed her to come directly to the maternity department. On arrival at the hospital, the nurse connected a fetal heart monitor to the patient and allowed her to listen to the baby's heartbeat. The patient went back home, reassured that her baby's heart was still beating in a normal rhythm. (Nurses and other health care workers who read this story will undoubtedly be concerned with the potential legal implications of the nurse's actions. Maternity departments are high-risk areas in terms of patient care and potential legal action. Health care providers must constantly use their judgment to balance quality-of-care issues with compassion for the person who is the patient. The nurse's actions in this case were based on practices that were appropriate at the time the care was provided, which would be different today.) In this particular instance, the patient ultimately completed her nursing education and chose to work in the hospital whose staff took care of her when she had no money to pay for medical care. In her eyes, the nurse represented the spirit or the culture of the hospital. She stated, "I never wanted to work anywhere else."

Policies and procedures are necessary to help employees make wise decisions. Written guidelines also help employees decide how to combine care for the person with care for the patient. Ulti-mately, it is the daily decisions of staff members throughout the organization that determine how the organization is viewed by the people they serve.

Case Study: A Culture Restructured at WakeMed

WakeMed* is a 716-bed, five-facility system located in Raleigh, North Carolina. In 1985, WakeMed began a strategic initiative to change the organization's corporate culture. The following infor-mation highlights the major steps that were taken to initiate the process and the structures that help the organization maintain its service culture.

In 1984, a community image analysis was completed, so that weaknesses in corporate goals could be identified and addressed. Following the community image survey, a guest relations program called "You Are the Difference" (YATD) was implemented. Train-ing for the management staff was implemented first, followed by training for the rest of the staff. The training was only the begin-ning of a long-term commitment to promoting a service-oriented organizational culture. Leaders knew at the outset that changing the culture would require a deeper commitment than guest rela-tions training alone.

Components of the Program

YATD is a comprehensive program designed to improve not only organizational success but also individual success. It is designed to educate employees about changes occurring in health care, services offered by WakeMed, personal and organizational values, continu-ous quality improvement (CQI), and customer service skills. In addi-tion to the vision, values, and services of the organization, employees

---

*Publications used for research for this case study are used with the permission of WakeMed, Raleigh, North Carolina.

also learn about revenue and expense categories, which promotes increased understanding of the financial goals of the organization. Skills that promote high-quality customer service and communication between coworkers are also included in the objectives.

A mandatory class is offered twice each month. The president of WakeMed attends each class to answer participants' questions. The distinctive feature that separates this class from educational programs that may be offered in other organizations is the follow-up that occurs outside of the classroom.

When employees were surveyed to determine how management could improve its commitment to quality, the suggestions they offered included greater trust between management and employees, management recognition of good work by departments and employees and sensitivity to staffing needs, and managers serving as role models and showing more concern for patients. Only 5 percent of employees responding to the survey asked for more money.

Recognition

A taskforce held workshops with approximately 300 employees to determine how employees wanted to be recognized. Some of the actions employees wanted recognition for included covering for other staff members, dealing effectively with difficult situations, personal and professional development, and exceeding standards. Employees indicated they would prefer recognition from colleagues or supervisors rather than upper management. Suggestions for recognition included many simple, inexpensive ideas, such as a letter in the employee's personnel file, a free lunch, or movie tickets. They also mentioned that a written thank-you note would be appreciated.

Following the employee workshops on recognition, a workshop for managers was conducted to share the results and discuss ways to address the employees' suggestions for recognition. Managers were provided with a recognition kit, which includes a questionnaire to help determine the kind of recognition their staff members would like.

The questionnaire includes demographic and lifestyle questions as well as open-ended questions about individual preferences for recognition. The information helps managers to give recognition in a way that does not embarrass employees who may prefer one-on-one thanks to being in a public spotlight. Rewards can also be consistent with employees' individual interests. Managers were also provided a recognition fund budget of $10 per employee, which they could use to recognize one employee, a team, or the entire department.

The Circle of Quality Service is the most significant customer service award. Employees are nominated by peers, and a committee of representative employees evaluates those nominated for the award. The winner receives a plaque that is later placed in the hospital lobby and a recognition pin, a focus article appears in the hospital newsletter, and a reception and an evening dance are held for employees. Winners of the award represent the top 1 percent of the organization.

Other Changes

WakeMed also revised its performance appraisal system to include 30 percent of its focus on quality service. Managers are encouraged to link a minimum of one job-specific standard to quality service. In some instances, up to 50 percent of an employee's pay could be related to quality service.

Another component of the YATD program at WakeMed includes senior management shadowing employees for a day. Twice each year, members of senior management work side by side with employees to learn firsthand the issues they face on a daily basis. The experience also allows the front-line employees to see the human side of senior management. The shadowing program is viewed as an enhancement of the employee recognition program. It provides an opportunity for senior management to truly understand and appreciate the work the employees do.

A President's Task Force evolved into the President's Quality Council to support the CQI efforts in the organization. Training and coaching for the quality improvement efforts are ongoing activities. Results achieved through the work of CQI teams are highlighted through storyboards and a CQI tracking index. A gain-sharing program was introduced to support quality improvement efforts that improve processes, reduce costs, or improve patient sat-isfaction. A monthly hospital publication, *The Wake Street Journal*, keeps employees informed of progress toward goals for the gain-sharing program. While there may be amendments to the program, one constant focus is patient satisfaction. If minimum levels are not achieved, there is no payout; when patient satisfaction is above tar-geted levels, the payout increases.

Ongoing Commitment

All employees participate in at least twenty hours of education on the YATD program following their ninety-day probation. Managers and supervisors receive additional training to ensure that commu-nication is consistent and that individual components of the pro-gram are administered consistently. One of the courses designed specifically for managers and supervisors teaches interviewing skills. The geographic area served by WakeMed has experienced a 1 or 2 percent unemployment rate for several years, which makes prese-lecting employees with the right skills and attitudes difficult. The YATD program has been constructed to instill the organization's values in employees through the initial orientation, the perfor-mance appraisal, and the gainsharing process. Continued commu-nication on progress toward goals is accomplished through the hospital's newsletter and the recognition program.

A description of the "You Are the Difference" program that was circulated to employees early in its development includes a quote by Tom Peters, a well-known author of business and man-agement books. The quote effectively summarizes the end result we all need to keep in mind as we set out to create structures that will support a high-performing organization. "The essence of excellence is the thousand concrete, minute-to-minute actions performed by everyone in an organization to keep a company on its course. Excellent companies are brilliant on just a few basics: behaving with courtesy toward customers, providing a continuous array of innovative products and services, and above all, gaining the commitment, ingenuity and energy of all employees."

Only a few elements of WakeMed's "You Are the Difference" program have been described here. Changing an organization's culture is a methodical, sometimes difficult and uncomfortable process. WakeMed began the program in 1985 and continues to evaluate individual components to make sure it is working as effectively as it should be.

References

Allerton, H. E. "Survey Says." *Training and Development*, Nov. 1998, 52(11).

Austin, N. K. "Killing Employees with Kindness." *Working Woman*, Jan. 1998.

Battistella, R., and Burchfield, D. "Defined Contribution: It's Inevitable." *Business and Health*, Nov. 1998.

Bond, J. T., Galinsky, E., and Swanberg, J. "Executive Summary." *The 1997 National Study of the Changing Workforce*. Publication no. W98-01. Families and Work Institute, 1998.

Cerrato, P. L. "Employee Health: Not Just a Fringe Benefit." *Business and Health*, Nov. 1995.

Cobb, J. C., Samuel, C. J., and Sexton, M. W. "Alignment and Strategic Change: A Challenge for Marketing and Human Resources." *Leadership & Organization Development Journal*, 1998, 19(1), 32–43.

Goetzel, R. Z., and others. "The Relationship Between Modifiable Health Risks and Health Care Expenditures: An Analysis of the Multi-Employer HERO Health Risk and Cost Database." *Journal of Environmental and Occupational Medicine*, Oct. 1998, 40(10).

Herman, R. E. "You've Got to Change to Retain." *HR Focus*, Sept. 1998, 75(9).

Kelley, S. "Some Steps for Dealing with High Employee Turnover." *Dallas Business Journal*, Sept. 4, 1998, 22(2).

Laabs, J. "They Want More Support—Inside and Outside of Work." *Workforce*, Nov. 1998, 77(11).

Woodward, N. H. "Add a Refreshing Touch to Benefit Programs." *HR Magazine*, Oct. 1998, 3(11).

Ziegler, J. "The Worker's Health: Whose Business Is it?" *Business and Health Special Report*, Dec. 1997.

Chapter Nine

Marketing

Although we recognize that employees have a significant impact on an organization's public image and relationships with existing patients (customer retention), a certain level of marketing is necessary to continue to attract new patients (customer acquisition). Marketing staff use organizational strategy to attract patients and develop appropriate new services to meet community needs. By working closely with human resources and operational departments, marketing staff will make sure that external and internal messages are compatible.

As we have stated earlier, we define marketing in a health care organization much more broadly than others in the industry. Marketing involves both the internal systems that affect the delivery of service to consumers and the traditionally defined arena of marketing—the external activities that result in leads and referrals to the organization: public relations, media relations, communications, and advertising.

We define marketing more broadly because the traditional, more limited definition that most health care administrators place on marketing—advertising—is the least effective, yet most costly, single function of marketing when viewed in light of research into how health care consumers make their decisions.

This chapter will focus on the less traditional functions of marketing, such as communicating patient expectations and perceptions to internal audiences, working with operational departments to make changes that will enhance patients' experiences, making sure that internal and external messages are congruent, and determining the long-term impact of marketing strategies. Some time will be spent on advertising, but we will not fully cover traditional public relations, publications, communications, media relations, and research aspects of the marketing function.

How Consumers Choose a Provider

The results of a survey by the National Research Corporation revealed that word of mouth is the most important factor influencing patients' selection of providers. Forty-seven percent of persons surveyed took the recommendation of a friend or family member. A strong general reputation was cited as important for 22 percent. Only 2 percent of respondents indicated advertising was the most significant factor in their decision making (Smoldt, 1998, p. 48).

According to a study that traced a company's reputation to the information source that caused the most uplift in favorable ratings, advertising was a distant last. Advertising accounted for only a 2 percent increase in positive reputation, compared with study participants' having used the company's product or service (12 percent) or knowing someone who worked there (30 percent) (Drennan, 1992). It seems a company's most important communications medium is its own employees.

Although advertising certainly increases awareness of health care services and providers and can further the general reputation of a facility, it does not have a significant impact on the immediate, actual decision for care. In fact, advertising can actually damage an organization's reputation when the actual patient experience is significantly different from the advertised experience or when the organization is not adequately prepared for the resulting increase in patient volume.

Perception Versus Reality

Each organization, whether in health care or another industry, has two images—the image the organization wishes to project to its customers or market and the image that its customers actually have of the organization. It would seem that health care institutions are having a significant identity crisis when we compare the two images.

When we look at health care organizations' mission statements, it is clear they exist to ease suffering, cure the sick, and prevent illness. They use words such as *care, compassion, respect, quality,* and *dignity.* They believe that they are providing high-quality care and that they truly care for the people who come to them.

Each day, each employee comes to work to do the best possible job he or she is capable of. (If managers don't believe that, they must believe the reverse—that employees make a conscious decision to come to work in order to make mistakes.) Patients expect that employees are capable of doing their jobs clinically as well as from a customer service standpoint. Patients depend on personal interaction with employees and physicians for the "care" in health care.

However, patients' perception of their health care organization may be significantly different from the one they have of the employees who care for them. As discussed in Chapter 4, the AHA's "Reality √ II" project showed clearly that the public can easily separate institutions from people. The people who work in hospitals are viewed as good and caring while the institution that surrounds them may or may not be viewed as positively.

The following are significant findings from "Reality √" and "Reality √ II" that bear repeating:

- The public perceives that organizational changes occur to enhance profits. Patients see little benefit to them, the care they receive, or their community from mergers and acquisitions.

- The patient's definition of quality is the nurse. Nurses have historically been viewed as patient advocates, but increasingly patients see no one as their advocate in an industry that is riddled with waste, fraud, and abuse.

- Patients develop an opinion about a hospital's image through their personal experiences, not from any promotional message. Patients also perceive advertising as driving up costs, especially at the expense of quality. They believe that if a hospital didn't spend as much on promotion, it would be able to afford more nurses to provide patient care.

- Even though patients believe we have the best technology and expertise in the world, they believe quality is declining and the reason is hospitals' emphasis on profits (American Hospital Association, 1996; American Hospital Association, 1997–1998).

The corporatization of health care strongly conflicts with people's perception of health care as more than just a business. Customers need to be reassured that they will get personal service. Employees who understand marketing and their role in working toward the hospital's goals are able to promote the positive aspects of the organization to patients rather than contribute to a negative perception such as that a clinical area is understaffed.

Fewer than half of Americans say they have "a great deal or quite a lot" of confidence in the health care system according to a survey conducted in 1998 by the Gallup Organization. Whereas 59 percent of the respondents had "a great deal or quite a lot" of confidence in organized religion, the highest institution ranked, only 40 percent had the same amount of confidence in the medical system (Gardner, 1998, p. 31).

Likewise, the "Eye on Patients" research study conducted by the American Hospital Association and the Picker Institute showed significant dissatisfaction with the health care industry. Respondents to this survey said that the good aspects of health care included the fact that doctors and nurses are courteous and that patients are treated with respect and they have their basic physical needs attended to. However, there were more negative than positive aspects to the health care industry. According to the patients surveyed: The system is a nightmare to navigate, with gatekeepers setting up too many barriers. Caregivers don't provide enough information, are not emotionally supportive, and don't involve patients in decisions about their care (Gardner, 1998, p. 33).

How can health care organizations combat these negative perceptions? In "Reality √," the AHA recommends that hospitals communicate to all audiences (employees, medical staff, volunteers, patients, and the community) in the language of quality of care, not the financial bottom line or corporate efficiencies. In fact, many hospital administrators will say that they do try to communicate in the language of quality. The problem is that health care organizations and their administrators speak a different language from consumers. We need to begin to speak in the consumer's language.

So often in health care, we say that patients don't know how to define quality of care, and that is part of the complexity and uniqueness of health care. In fact, patients do know how to define quality and they have been telling us for years—we just haven't been listening. We have been trying to tell the patient how to define quality rather than listening to their definition because we believe we know more than they do about health care.

When we begin to listen to how the patient defines quality, we can begin to provide care in the way they wish to receive it, not the way it is most convenient for us to provide it. Patients certainly expect the type of "quality of care" health care organizations define—the latest technology, technical expertise, and positive clinical outcomes. In fact, they consider that type of quality a given.

But patients don't always define quality by whether they or a loved one gets well (or doesn't get sick). Despite the best efforts, patients get ill and patients die. It is an inevitable and unavoidable fact of life. Patients define quality by how they are treated as individuals, the respect they are given by health care providers, how much they are involved in the discussion of treatment options, and how their families are treated. They define quality by whether the doctors, nurses, and other staff genuinely seem to care about what the patient is experiencing. They define quality by whether the doctors, nurses, and other staff treat the patient as an individual or as "the gallbladder in 215."

Quality of care cannot be communicated with words on a mission statement, in a meeting, on a chart, through an advertisement, or in a brochure. The type of quality of care patients want can only be communicated between one employee and one patient at a time or one doctor and one patient at a time. And it is the only thing that will bridge the confidence gap and rebuild the trust that patients once had in health care institutions. The thing that will differentiate one provider from another is service.

Internal Communications

Internal communications from a marketing perspective are generally considered to be employee newsletters, the most common connecting factor between marketing and human resources departments. But internal communications need to be broader than that in order to make sure that employees are truly educated on the organization's mission, vision, values, patient expectations, and their role in marketing the organization. Not only is the message important, so is the medium.

The first messages that need to be communicated consistently, frequently, and in a variety of styles are the mission, vision, and values of the organization. In fact, Kotter (1996, p. 9) says that under-communicating the vision is one of the most significant mistakes any organization can make. "Major change is usually impossible unless most employees are willing to help, often to the point of making short-term sacrifices. But people will not make sacrifices, even if they are unhappy with the status quo, unless they think the potential benefits of change are attractive and unless they really believe that a transformation is possible. Without credible communication, and a lot of it, employee's hearts and minds are never captured."

According to Kotter, there are three common patterns of ineffective communication that develop during stable periods. The first is using only a small portion of the available organizational media—usually a couple of meetings or the company newsletter once or twice—to announce the new initiative. The second pattern occurs when the vision is communicated more generally to employees, but not vocally supported by managers. The third, and more deadly, pattern occurs when the vision is widely communicated but is sabotaged by key, visible individuals within the organization who continue to act within the old vision and are not forced to accept negative consequences for their nonsupportive actions.

The second message that needs to be consistently communicated internally is patient expectations. Marketing departments are often the administrators of the patient satisfaction program and therefore have a wealth of knowledge about what makes patients satisfied or dissatisfied. The marketing staff are also involved in both formal market research (surveys and focus groups) and informal research (involvement in community activities in which they learn about public perceptions). Marketing staff need to constantly and consistently communicate patient expectations to the organization as a whole, to individual departments, and to the human resources department so that improvements and appropriate hiring decisions can be made and patient expectations met.

Employee Communications

Employee communications are important because a motivated, educated, knowledgeable workforce can better achieve corporate goals, better serve as front-line ambassadors, and implement change initiatives more effectively and more quickly. However, the definition of employee communications needs to be expanded from the traditional employee newsletter to a variety of other communication strategies.

Internal communication begins at orientation, as outlined in Chapter 7. Employees are given information about the organization's mission, vision, and values and about important issues such as customer service. This may also be an appropriate time to introduce the concept that although there is a marketing department within the organization, marketing is the responsibility of each employee. Such issues as what marketing is, how individual employees market services, and responsibilities of the marketing department could easily be covered in thirty minutes within new employee orientation.

How employees receive information is just as important as the message itself. Pairing a new employee with a preceptor or other mentor, as suggested in Chapter 7, is an excellent way to provide face-to-face communication opportunities about organizational and customer expectations. This allows opportunities for an employee to ask specific questions about items he or she has read in policies and procedures manuals as part of orientation.

The employee newsletter—the main method of formal communication within organizations—is an effective tool to communicate a consistent message to a large number of people in an efficient manner. Employees who pick up the newsletter all receive the same information delivered in the same way at the same time, which makes it an attractive medium for management.

However, a printed newsletter is not the form of communication preferred by employees. Employees prefer verbal communication directly from their supervisor, with printed material serving as a backup. Regular, scheduled departmental staff meetings or other forms of individual or group discussion with direct supervisors are much preferred.

Very often, however, managers are not prepared to communicate directly with employees, especially on sensitive issues. Communicating with employees in their preferred style may require training supervisory and management staff to help them understand employees' needs, different communication styles, how to listen, various employee groups' sensitivity to issues, how to communicate a potentially negative message, and how to role-play questions and answers. Marketing communications specialists can assist training and development specialists in teaching supervisors and managers to be better communicators.

The communication that occurs between supervisors and employees can be reinforced through the various training programs in which employees participate. If customer service is a major organizational initiative, it can be stressed in training programs throughout the organization, even in clinical or technical training sessions. If the organization is undergoing a significant change initiative, every training session should emphasize how this training fits into the overall strategy. Staff development professionals can help employees

- Understand their changing role within the organization
- Learn what additional skills they need to acquire to continue their growth
- Understand the organization's mission and how their job relates to it

Another form of printed communication directed toward employees is motivational posters. Although these can occasionally present a positive message to employees, frequently they backfire because employees view them as overly preachy and being "talked down to." One health care organization subscribed to a series of motivational posters with excellent photography and subtle messages. The posters were changed weekly and were enjoyed by the employees; many called the marketing office when the new poster went up asking for it when the week was over. Management believed that had employees not noticed whether the posters were changed, the money would have been wasted on the project.

A major hotel operated by a national chain reminded employees of the importance of their job, regardless of the situation or their personal mood, by hanging a shiny brass plaque on the employee-only side of the door to the main lobby simply announcing that employees were about to enter "Center Stage."

Communication with Other Internal Audiences

Unlike other industries, which may have limited internal audiences, health care organizations have a variety of internal audiences with whom to communicate. Physicians, physician office staff, volunteers, and donors can be considered internal audiences and should be included in major communication strategies. In some cases, these audiences receive the same printed communications as employees but rarely receive the same personal contact, which can be a serious omission.

Because of the close working relationship between clinical employees and physicians, employees are frequently the primary face-to-face communication medium for physicians. This is another reason it is extremely important for all employees to clearly understand organizational objectives, their role in organizational strategy, and the importance of organizational objectives so they can clearly communicate them to physicians, patients, and their contacts within the community. Well-informed employees can communicate the organization's goals and objectives and replace misconceptions and misunderstandings with accurate information.

New Ideas

It is easy to continually rely on traditional internal communication media. However, health care organizations need to regularly introduce new communication tools like the following in order to make sure that they reach all their audiences in the best possible way.

- The introduction of Intranet and company e-mail systems offers some opportunity for brief messages to be placed on "hello" or "sign-on" screens.
- Screen savers can be programmed into networked computers and changed on a regular basis.
- Informal opportunities for supervisory, management, and executive employees to meet with direct patient care employees can be created through scheduled meetings or simply by encouraging them to eat meals with patient care employees on a regular basis. This sounds like such a simple action, but visibility and accessibility of members of the management team, especially in a mostly social setting, can have a significant positive impact on employee morale.

- Hold a "marketing fair" for employees, medical staff, and physician office staff each year, similar to a human resources benefits fair. The purpose of the fair would be to showcase the various clinical services the hospital offers, as well as the community services available (speakers' bureau, health fairs, specialty items, brochures, and so on).

External Communications

The largest amount of time and money spent by hospital marketing departments is for the following external communications to retain and attract customers:

- Brochures, newsletters, magazines, annual reports, and other printed materials
- Advertising
- Web site development and maintenance
- Attendance at exhibits and other events

Because of the amount of resources placed into these external efforts, it is vitally important that marketing staff understand organizational goals. Knowing who the audience is, the best way to reach it, and the return on investment for each promotional effort means that resources are placed in those media that provide the most value for both the audience and the organization. It also ensures that a promotional campaign fits into the organizational mission rather than simply being a reaction to competitive forces or industry trends.

The first step after incorporating the organization's mission, vision, and values is to identify customers and the services they require. A facility's location and the demographics of the immediate area will in part direct the type of services it offers. A hospital located in a growing population area attracting young families will need to offer excellent obstetric and pediatric services. A hospital located in a retirement community will need to offer services for an elderly population, such as orthopedics, oncology, and internal medicine.

Once the audience is defined, the second step is to develop the right message to reach it. A consistent message that incorporates individual service lines will be more effective than each individual service line having a separate identity.

The third step is to make sure that the external message matches internal and external attitudes, perceptions, and reality. This means that not only does the external message have to closely resemble what the patient's actual experience is likely to be, the external audience has to believe that it will match. If a hospital traditionally known as a general primary care provider begins promoting itself as the leader in a particular area of clinical expertise, it will probably meet with some skepticism. Consumers generally have three or four national and one or two local clinical leaders in mind. Patients understand that every organization cannot be the leader in every clinical area.

Internal audiences must also be aware of external messages so that they are not surprised by the message or its timing and frequency. Customers can be frustrated when they call for specific information only to be transferred to various individuals who are not able to meet their needs.

Employee recruitment materials should also provide consistent internal and external messages. Employment ads need to be consistent with the theme of other institutional advertising and promotion efforts and the message needs to be consistent with employees' actual work experience.

Consider the reaction of prospective, as well as current, employees to the following ad:

> Blank Hospital has improved on near perfection. In one of the most stress-free settings in America, set against endless, rolling hills and lush forests, health care professionals will find paradise. For their careers, that is. We offer comprehensive and progressive professional growth programs, competitive salaries, and good benefits. Explore

the opportunities with us and discover just how perfect your life—
and your career—can be.

Current and prospective employees understand that perfection
does not exist in any employment situation. The question for this
particular hospital is whether or not the real employment situation
matches this preferred image.

How to Communicate

In 1991, the Gallup Organization conducted a telephone survey of
100,000 people for Inforum, a health care planning and marketing
information company. The survey found that 60 percent of consumers would prefer to receive their health care information via
direct mail. Newspaper and television were preferred by 6 percent
each, and 17 percent preferred "other," which could include hospital
publications such as brochures and magazines ("Data Watch," 1992).

However the way health care institutions actually communicate
with their external audience is quite different, according to a 1996
survey conducted by ORC Health Care. Forty-three percent of
health care advertising communications are by newspapers or magazines, with 14 percent by radio, 12 percent by direct mail, and 11
percent by television. Yellow pages were represented in the survey
results at 11 percent, other media at 5 percent, and bus/billboards at
4 percent (Opinion Research Corporation International, 1996).

This discrepancy between consumers' preferences and marketers' actions clearly shows that marketing professionals need to
pay better attention to their forms of communication.

The Costs and Benefits of Advertising

In 1997, hospitals and hospital systems spent $2.4 billion on market-
ing. Slightly more than half of that ($1.3 billion) was spent on adver-
tising, according to ORC. Overall, hospitals spent roughly $1,100
per licensed bed in 1996 for advertising (Bellandi, 1998, p. 82).

These numbers help explain why patients believe that advertising and marketing drive up the cost of health care. When an advertising campaign is developed to meet clear organizational goals and is coordinated with other internal and external communications, it can be very effective in delivering the organization's message. Too often, however, advertising campaigns are developed in response to external pressures, not organizational objectives. These advertising-war campaigns are the ones that are perceived negatively by patients as contributing to increased costs.

Positive Promotion

Market research has shown that because of the personal nature of health care, the most effective organizational ambassadors are employees. But it would be impossible for a hospital's employees to talk face-to-face with every member of the community the hospital serves, which is why advertising and other external promotional efforts are necessary. Those can also be extremely effective, but only when the message matches the actual patient experience.

Remember the lessons from the "Reality √" projects:

- People believe their real experiences rather than advertising, but they respond positively to health care advertising that provides useful information about maintaining their health or when it reinforces the personal care they received.

- Twenty-two percent of consumers choose a health care provider on the basis of a strong general reputation which can, in part, be influenced by advertising.

- Advertising only brings in "leads" to an organization. The final and ultimate decision of image and reputation is made by the patient based on the relationship with individual employees involved in the patient's care (American Hospital Association, 1996; American Hospital Association, 1997–1998).

Written promotional materials (advertising, brochures, newsletters, and magazines) can multiply word-of-mouth messages. When an organization can use patient endorsements in its promotional materials it provides an opportunity for hundreds or thousands to hear what might have only been heard by a few people on a personal basis.

Advertising also builds awareness of and excitement about the services your organization offers, especially among employees. Increased employee morale is often a by-product of a promotion campaign that positively represents the hospital. Employees are proud to work for an organization that is represented in that manner.

Not only is it important to retain existing patients through positive patient contact experiences, it is important to attract new patients. General media advertising and promotional efforts such as newcomer programs direct new residents to your services and introduce them to your capabilities.

A consistent promotional campaign that includes advertising, public relations, publications, and media relations can build a brand identity among your community members so they begin to recognize and become familiar with your organization's image and identity.

Marketing as an Operational Support

There are times when promoting a service is not the best immediate alternative. In this type of situation, the marketing and human resources staff can work with operational departments to facilitate changes that need to be made in order to improve a service before it is promoted.

Marketing directors will be familiar with the following scenario: The director of a department notices a downward spiral in patient visits and admission. She and the chief physician make a visit to the marketing director and say, "We need to advertise our department to generate more business." or "We need a brochure for our department to hand out to patients."

The easiest answer for the marketing director is to add this request onto the department's "to do" list. However, a better long-term alternative for the organization would be to investigate the root causes or trends involved in the decrease. Often, this type of investigation may reveal changes in insurance coverage, business climate, market demographics, or patient perceptions that simple promotional activities would not affect.

Declines in patient volume often require working with the operational manager to obtain the resources to change certain factors within the hospital's control. These factors may include physical changes to the department to improve patient flow, changes in employee responsibilities to increase efficiency, or working with employees to make the best of less-than-ideal physical facilities. It could also include working closely and personally with external groups to modify market situations or community perceptions.

Marketing and human resources staff are well equipped to use patient satisfaction surveys, employee and patient focus groups, other external market research, community assessments, job descriptions and job inventories, and group facilitation techniques to work through issues. Once this process is completed, the volume may adjust to its goal level or there may still be a need to promote the service.

A promotion needs to be closely coordinated with the operational department in order to make adjustments when it is too successful and begins to outstrip the staff's ability to meet the demand. This occurred to Sinai Hospital of Baltimore when it opened its new emergency department—ER-7—in 1997.

The previous emergency department had been designed and constructed in the late 1970s to accommodate up to 40,000 annual patient visits. In 1997, that ED served more than 54,000 patients. Staff members from the department of strategic development (now the integrated marketing, communications, community services, and development department) were involved in the development of ER-7 from the very beginning. The multidisciplinary task force studied other facilities that were customer service leaders and surveyed former and potential ED patients to get their input into the new facility (a key factor in the new department's success). Two important customer concerns were addressed in ER-7: reduced waiting time and more privacy for the patient and family.

> The response to the ER-7 advertising campaign was so overwhelming that visits to the center far exceeded expectations. This was a positive outcome from a marketing perspective, but from an operational perspective, it presented a challenge for the ER-7 staff. ER-7's initial staffing was based on about a 10 percent increase over previous rates. During the first few weeks of the marketing and public relations campaign, ER visits were up as much as 35 percent. The ER-7 management team requested that the marketing plan be scaled back to allow time to hire and train additional staff. The campaign was pulled back, and six weeks later, the advertising resumed according to plan [Bloom, Warns, and Giller, 1998, p. 6].

Close contact between marketing and operational departments will help ensure that trends are closely monitored and small adjustments in promotional efforts can be made before situations become disastrous.

Other Marketing Functions

Although we have focused primarily on the promotional aspects of marketing within this chapter, there are other significant marketing capabilities that can assist operational departments in achieving their goals.

Through primary and secondary market research, the marketing staff can provide operational departments with the data they need to make decisions. This includes patient satisfaction surveys, which are often, but not always, conducted through the marketing department.

The development of new services is also a major responsibility of marketing staff. By conducting the basic market research on trends, patient satisfaction levels, and consumer preferences, marketing staff can analyze data to help operational departments make decisions on new services or develop ideas for new services. This support can include the development of a business plan and/or a marketing plan. Human resources staff also need to be involved in new service development because the addition of a new service has obvious staffing implications.

Customer Satisfaction

As stated earlier, marketing and human resources staff both have the capability and responsibility to help develop a culture of customer service excellence within the organization. Together, these two departments can help invest in the organization's intellectual capital by placing less emphasis on market share and beating the competition and more emphasis on creating relationships with patients, encouraging continuing use of services, and creating greater value for customers.

The key is in learning how to motivate staff to be responsive to the critical factors that influence patients' overall satisfaction with their health care experience. This can be done through skill training and behavioral coaching based on organizational values and patient expectations.

The skill training and behavioral coaching should help employees understand those expectations of the health care experience that are most important to the patient and how to translate them into behavior that makes a positive impact on the patient.

Patient satisfaction survey company Press, Ganey Associates (1997) analyzed more than a million patient surveys conducted at its client hospitals over a 12-month period from 1995 to 1996. It was able to identify ten issues most closely correlated with a patient's likelihood of recommending that hospital to a friend or family member:

- Staff sensitivity to the inconvenience that health problems and hospitalization can cause

- Overall cheerfulness of the hospital
- Staff concern about patient privacy
- Amount of attention paid to special or personal needs
- Degree to which nurses took patients' health problems seriously
- Technical skill of nurses
- Nurses' attitude on the phone
- Degree to which the nurses kept patients adequately informed about tests, treatment, and equipment
- Friendliness of nurses
- Promptness of nurses in responding to call button

Customer satisfaction training at an individual hospital can incorporate this information with feedback from other sources to customize the training to an organization's own customer base and market.

One-to-One Marketing

One-to-one marketing has been a popular topic in health care marketing over the past few years. It is a challenge to create a one-to-one marketing program in health care similar to retail programs because of the confidential nature of health care. Hospitals that choose to implement such programs need to carefully think through the various implications before proceeding.

Marketing promotions are essential tools for health care organizations, but relationships are not built on the basis of direct mail or advertisements. They are built on familiarity, frequent contact, trust, and shared interest. Health care is ultimately about relationships: of patient and physician, of patient and nurse, of medical staff and administration, of employee and supervisor, of marketing and human resources. Relationships that can become significant long-term relationships are made each day. A patient may become a volunteer, a donor, an employee, an ally, a supplier of feedback, a word-of-mouth ambassador, or all of the above. As you develop these relationships, you build the organization's success, achieve its goals, and, at the same time, meet patient expectations.

The Long-Term Impact of Marketing Communications

Marketing and human resources efforts need to be seen as long-term investments, although there are some excellent examples of immediate results that can be achieved through marketing. An advertising campaign intended to change an organization's image may gain the attention of former, current, or prospective patients, but immediate results are not always possible. People don't usually need health care services as often as they purchase food, a car, or even a house. It may be several weeks, months, or even years before the consumer needs health care services and will then be in a position to compare the advertised service with the real service.

This long-term view could have an impact on the way the financial impact of marketing communications is viewed, according to MacStravic (1998, p. 53). "The long-term impact of marketing communications has traditionally been overlooked in the way accountants and financial officers look at marketing expenditures, insisting on treating them as expenses when they occur, rather than 'capital' investments to be amortized over longer periods. This myopic view hampers the planning and execution of marketing efforts that will not pay off sufficiently in the same fiscal year to which expenditures will be charged."

When marketing is viewed from a broader perspective, it can be seen that organizational goals drive market research, which drives operational support, customer satisfaction efforts, and new service development. These are then supported by the traditional marketing functions of advertising and promotion.

Case Study: The 90-Day Checkup
of Baptist Hospital of Pensacola

It is a cliché these days to say that the best way to satisfy your customers is to satisfy your employees. Like favoring motherhood and apple pie, it's a hard thesis to argue against. But as a manager, how do you get started? How do you actually change a company's culture? And how do you know if you're succeeding?

Quinton Studer, president of Baptist Hospital Inc., in Pensacola, Florida, came up with the answers to these questions. He arrived in Pensacola in 1996 from a stint as senior vice president at Holy Cross Hospital in Chicago and has spent the past several years developing a system to improve both patient and employee satisfaction.

Surprisingly, the model is based on his years as a special-education teacher. "Maximizing an organization's ability is similar to maximizing a child's potential," Studer says. "The first step is to diagnose the situation and then set achievable goals. The higher the goals, the closer the student—or organization—comes to reaching full potential. Every 90 days the teacher does an individual education plan to ensure that all resources directed to the child are aligned with the goals. And at the end of a year, old goals are reassessed and new ones are set."

While that's the basic plan, Studer has refined his system over the years and brought it to the point where it is replicable not only in other hospitals but in any service business.

When Studer arrived, Baptist's admissions were flat and patient satisfaction as measured by a national survey was slightly below average. After just two years—in an industry in which admissions are staying the same or going down—Baptist's admissions were up 8.3 percent. Outpatient volume was up 33 percent. As for patient satisfaction, Baptist ranked number two in the country for all hospitals and number one for hospitals with more than 100 beds. Employee satisfaction had improved 30 percent and physician satisfaction had risen from 72.4 percent to 81.3 percent. Job turnover for nurses went from 30 percent to 18 percent. *Inc.* magazine senior editor Nancy J. Lyons (1999) queried Studer about Baptist's cultural turnaround.

Lyons: Changing a culture seems more than ambitious—it's an absolutely daunting idea. Yet you seem to have accomplished a great deal in a very short time at Baptist. How did you get started?

Studer: We decided we had to have a measurable service goal. I believe you have to measure what's important to you, and that you have to have some means of comparison. If a company can't afford an outside group to do a survey, which I strongly recommend, it should develop its own tool. So, first of all, we met with all the employees and talked about why the hospital exists, what our purpose is. They said that they wanted to be the best. Becoming the employer of choice also became a goal at Baptist.

Lyons: So you started out measuring patient satisfaction?

Studer: Yes. We use a large patient-satisfaction-measurement company that can compare us with at least 500 hospitals across the country. We send a survey to every patient. The results help us set specific goals. They also give us an opportunity to recognize employees who receive positive comments on the survey.

Lyons: OK, so you know where you stand from the survey, and you know where you want to go. But up to now, nothing has changed, right? It seems that this would be where most CEOs would get stuck.

Studer: What we do next is the number one thing companies just don't want to spend money on: middle-management development. We take every one of our leaders—nurse managers, supervisors, and department heads—off-site for two days every ninety days. We also have employee forums every ninety days and survey employees on their attitudes toward their supervisors. Our employees knew their supervisors hadn't had any "real" training, but we also let them know it's an organizational issue—not their supervisor's issue—to provide development. We call it leadership muscle building. That's what my whole job is about. Accountability, by the way, is key.

Lyons: What do you mean by accountability? Who's accountable to whom and for what?

Studer: All our leaders get "report cards" every ninety days. That's how we align behaviors to our goals and how we can reward objectively, which takes politics out of the game. A typical person in our organization will have four measurements. One is customer service, which we measure against our goal, which is to be in the top 1 percent of hospitals in the country. All the employees know what will satisfy our customers and where our weaknesses lie, because they know the results of the patient-satisfaction survey. The second measurement looks at efficiency: how long patients are in their units per diagnosis. The third one is expense management: how well they're managing expenses. The fourth thing we're measuring this year is turnover. Everyone's got a turnover goal based on his or her unit and its past history.

Lyons: When you say everyone has a turnover goal, does that include top managers as well?

Studer: Yes, our vice-presidents also have their own report cards and are measured on the same four categories as middle managers are. Twenty percent of my incentive compensation is based on employee turnover. That gets my attention.

Lyons: What sorts of things do you do to slow down the turnover?

Studer: We used the same sort of survey tool to measure employee satisfaction as we'd used to measure customer satisfaction. We found out that the biggest thing that bugged our employees was that their evaluations were late. They want feedback. Employees also want supervisors who accept their input with respect and appreciation. They want to know about matters that affect them. So we measured. And we set goals for where we wanted to be. We took all our leaders off-site and taught them how to present the survey data. Then we did ninety-day work plans with employees, itemizing what we were going to change in the workplace to make it better. Then we measured again, and rewarded and recognized our accomplishments. I believe in strong rewards and recognition.

Lyons: What sort of rewards and recognition?

Studer: Every company has outstanding people. We make heroes of them. One of our nurses, Cyd Cadena, called up a lady who had been hospitalized to see how she was doing at home. She was in a wheelchair, and she was depressed because she didn't have a wheelchair ramp. The family was so busy working on home health care and a whole bunch of other things that they didn't get a chance to put in a ramp. Well, Cyd called our plant-management person, Don Swartz. And guess what Don did? He built a ramp. Don didn't ask, "Can I do it?" I found out about it because the patient called me. Now we tell that story all over the whole organization. What did we tell our people it was OK to do? Break a few rules. Take a few risks. Don is a star. You have to celebrate your legends.

Lyons: Tell us some of the other things that Baptist Hospital is doing to make it "the employer of choice."

Studer: Anybody who's ever been in a hospital knows we lose stuff. Patients complain about lost glasses, lost dentures, lost robes. And we ask dumb questions like "Are you sure you brought them with you?" "Are you sure your family doesn't have them?" "Why don't we wait and maybe they'll show up after discharge?" That leaves the employee dealing with a very unhappy patient, who doesn't get a check from us until three weeks after he or she has left the hospital. Today we have $250 available for any employee in the hospital to access on the spot to cover the cost of a patient's lost glasses or whatever.

We had a crazy rule in housekeeping that bugged the employees. Only our housekeepers were allowed to have housekeeping supplies. So if a nurse on a unit spilled something, and the unit coordinator or nurse wanted to clean it up, he or she couldn't. Instead, people spent twenty minutes saying, "Watch out! Don't step there. We've called housekeeping." Why weren't we allowing our staff to have housekeeping supplies in their unit? Trust. They might have taken them home. We didn't know we were this crazy until we started asking the employees what they needed.

Lyons: Any other advice for CEOs on getting employees to buy into their ideas for change?

Studer: Well, you have to really believe in what you're doing. When I got to Baptist, I said, "We're going to be the best hospital in the country," and somebody said, "Quint, you mean county." I said, "No, I mean country." You have to decide what you want to do, act on that decision, and look at the results. Then you get understanding. Sometimes we just have to get people to change their behavior and then they'll understand what we're after.

I'll give you an example. We have a rule at Baptist: We don't point. We think it's rude. We take people to where they're going. The other day I got a nice letter from a patient who said what impressed him the most was that when he walked into the hospital, somebody took him to where he needed to go. I don't know who it was, but whoever it was was a caregiver at that moment. Now, Bob Harriman, the VP of ambulatory care—he told me this later—thought it was a dumb idea. He didn't have time to guide people through the hospital. But I had to believe that if you actually take patients to where they need to go, it'll make a difference in how they view the hospital. We made the decision that's what we were going to do, and basically forced it for a while. The second time Harriman took someone to where that person was going, he understood and became a believer.

So sometimes we've just got to get people to do the behavior and then trust that they'll understand it afterward and become believers. You can get so hung up on getting everybody to understand what you're doing and why you're doing it that it never happens. Don't overworry about understanding. It will come, provided you act.*

---

*Republished with permission of *Inc.* magazine, Goldhirsh Group, Inc., 38 Commercial Wharf, Boston, MA 02110. "The 90-Day Checkup," Nancy Lyons, March 1999. Reproduced by permission of the publisher via Copyright Clearance Center, Inc.

References

American Hospital Association. "Reality √: Public Perceptions of Health Care and Hospitals." Chicago: American Hospital Association, 1996.

American Hospital Association, "Reality √ II: More Public Perceptions of Health Care and Hospitals." Chicago: American Hospital Association, 1997–1998.

Bellandi, D. "Big Ad Bucks." *Modern Healthcare*, Apr. 6, 1998.

Bloom, J., Warns, M., and Giller, D. "Strategy and Innovation in ER Services." *Spectrum*, Society for Healthcare Strategy and Market Development, Nov./Dec. 1998.

"Data Watch: Survey—Consumers Prefer Direct-Mail Campaigns." *Hospitals*, Apr. 20, 1992.

Drennan, D. *Transforming Company Culture*. New York: McGraw-Hill, 1992.

Gardner, J. "Dueling for Public Support." *Modern Healthcare*, Aug. 17, 1998.

Kotter, J. P. *Leading Change*. Boston, Mass.: Harvard Business School Press, 1996.

Lyons, N. J. "The 90-Day Checkup." *Inc.*, Goldhirsh Group, Inc., Mar. 1999.

MacStravic, S. "Marketing Myopia." *Healthcare Forum Journal*, Sept./Oct. 1998.

Opinion Research Corporation International. "1996 National Hospital Marketers' Survey." Evanston, Ill.: Opinion Research Corporation International, 1996.

Press, Ganey Associates, Inc. "One Million Patients Have Spoken: Who Will Listen?" News release, Jan. 10, 1997.

Smoldt, R. K. "Turn Word of Mouth into a Marketing Advantage." *Healthcare Forum Journal*, Sept./Oct. 1998.

Chapter Ten

Beginning the Change Process

In the opening of his novel *Something of Value*, Ruark (1955) cites an African Basuto proverb: "If a man does away with his traditional way of living and throws away his good customs, he had better first make certain that he has something of value to replace them." In health care as well as in other businesses, employees are challenged to move forward with sweeping changes without the benefit of knowing whether the old familiar processes will indeed be replaced with something of value. A common reaction to change is fear that something is being lost or thrown away. Leaders who are skilled in coaching people through the process of change will be vital to the continued success of organizations working toward new visions.

Many models have been designed to help people understand the attitudes and behavior associated with change. Familiarity with typical stages of change and corresponding behavior can help leaders understand their own personal reactions and also how to help others in the organization adjust to change. Promoting successes that occur during times of transition can help employees enjoy the journey rather than simply enduring it. According to consultants Townsend and Gebhardt (1997, pp. 22–23), "making change possible while maintaining individual and corporate sanity is one of the primary responsibilities of leadership. At any time, leaders are responsible for establishing an environment in which others can reach their full potential while simultaneously completing the job."

Following are some guidelines they suggest leaders should follow to help make change exciting rather than frightening:

- *Never institute change for the sake of change.* If a perception exists that a change is based on a fad, trust between management and members of the organization may be destroyed.

- *Prepare the environment.* Communicate with people about the change and allow them to be a part of the process.

- *Show concern for both projects and people.* The military defines the top two goals of leadership as accomplishing the mission and taking care of people. Put a buffer between people when necessary and avoid making changes that will put people in an impossible situation.

- *Know your people and demand the best from them.* People will live up or down to expectations. Work to understand the capabilities of all members of the team.

- *Share knowledge.* People are capable of contributing their best effort only when they know where things stand and in what direction the organization is moving.

- *Recognize accomplishments.* People are appreciative of thank-you's and they are more likely to increase their commitment if their efforts are acknowledged.

Leading People Through the Process of Change

The initial reaction of most people to the idea of linking human resources and marketing tends to be confusion, curiosity, and, eventually, an acknowledgment that it may indeed have some merit. The part of us that thinks in a traditional organizational-chart kind of way may wonder how or why these two areas should be linked together. In reality, many examples of successfully linking the two functions do not include a formal merger between the two areas.

In most of the case studies presented, success was achieved by enhancing the communication between the people carrying out the two functions and focusing on areas of agreement. Less important than the location of positions or departments on the organizational chart is a common understanding of the strategic goals and the methods that will enable employees to effectively contribute to the achievement of those goals.

A combination of broad philosophical ideas and hands-on or how-to approaches has been included to provide various avenues for discussion. A vision cannot become a reality without the tools needed to implement the plans that are designed to achieve the vision.

To summarize, the steps we have outlined in this book to effectively link the human resources and marketing functions include:

- Reviewing where health care has been (as a discipline; as an individual organization)

- Defining the roles involved in creating and carrying out the mission, vision, and values of the organization

- Evaluating the big picture to determine how individual strategies fit

- Developing employees to assist in the linking of the human resources and marketing functions

- Defining which employees are right for the organization

- Hiring the right people or developing skills in people who possess many of the desirable qualities that promote the organization's values

- Providing both training and development opportunities for employees

- Reviewing structures that help support the philosophies presented

- Marketing internally and externally

The examples and case studies presented in the preceding chapters contain some common themes. These include creating a vision, defining measurable goals, and involving employees in making decisions. Many vision or mission statements are built on the concept of being the best or providing the highest quality. The difficulty is in defining "best" and "quality" in ways that are measurable and understood by the people implementing the business plan.

"Being 'in between' the old and the new feels like failure, like nothing is right or sacred. This will change" (James, 1997, p. 26). Ironically, the nature of change provides us with assurance that as old familiar processes are left behind, the awkward transition between the old and the new is also a temporary situation.

Report from the Future

Well-known health care futurist Leland Kaiser began a presentation to a group of health care leaders with a statement about the future of health care. He made reference to traveling to the future and finding nothing there, because we have not yet created it. The concept is both frightening and exciting. There is comfort in familiar day-to-day tasks, even if they are not the right tasks that will lead us to greater success. The excitement associated with new opportunities is viewed as a motivator for some people and a matter of wishful thinking to others. We sometimes think it would be much easier to accomplish sweeping organizational changes if we could start over completely and rebuild the entire organization. In reality, leaders must find ways to promote new ways of thinking in the midst of carrying out established organizational processes.

The entire health care provider team will need to understand how to think in the "future tense." James (1997, pp. 26–31), a cultural anthropologist, has identified steps to help accomplish this task. Her recommendations are not step-by-step tasks that can be incorporated into a rigid format. They present an opportunity to evaluate personal philosophies of how we approach the future.

- *See with new eyes.* Work to develop a sense of perspective that helps to sort out the positives and the negatives of a new situation and better understand how all of the pieces fit together.
- *Recognize the future.* Study changes in the health care markets to better judge whether a new idea is a fad or an indication of true and lasting change.

- *Harness the power of myths and symbols*. Recognize the myths that have existed for so long within an organization or within the larger health care system that employees have come to accept them as fact.

- *Speed up your response time*. Be aware of barriers that will slow forward movement; some of these barriers include fear of loss, waiting for others to change, lack of confidence, and the need for control.

- *Understand the past to know the future*. Create a realistic future based on where the organization has been.

- *Do more with less*. This is perhaps the least favorite piece of advice for health care workers who are accustomed to working without adequate numbers of staff. This suggestion refers to the process of truly empowering employees to make suggestions and improvements.

- *Master new forms of intelligence*. Create a new vision of intelligence; one that includes both right-brain and left-brain thinking patterns.

- *Profit from diversity*. Cultural beliefs may cause separation of people who could potentially benefit the organization.

Learn from the Best

Once the leaders of an organization have agreed on the direction, specific steps to achieve the vision must be defined. An important prerequisite to making change is to put together a "fact base." The combination of the fact base and an understanding of the organization's values can provide the tools that are needed for employees to make wise decisions. The criteria for earning the Malcolm Baldrige Quality award provide a benchmark for many organizations. The award is one of the best recognized symbols of excellence in business.

Following is a list of ten core values that are the foundation of the Malcolm Baldrige Quality award:

1. *Customer-driven quality.* The customer ultimately decides how well the organization performs. It is essential to listen and respond to dissatisfied customers while continuing to keep loyal customers satisfied with the service they receive.

2. *Continuous improvement and learning.* The organization grows stronger and smarter by continuously evaluating and improving its processes.

3. *Management by fact.* Data adds vital hard facts to intuition. All employees need to be aware of the data that are available to them in making daily decisions about the work they do.

4. *Employee participation and development.* The people who do the work should make the majority of the decisions about how the work is done. It is vital to provide employees with the data they need, as mentioned in the previous point.

5. *Fast response.* Continuously analyze work processes to determine whether they can be completed more efficiently. Preventing problems and providing high-quality services may require an investment upfront, but the cost will most likely be less than the cost of correcting problems later.

6. *Long-range view of the future.* Establish measurable goals to determine progress toward long-range goals and communicate progress to employees regularly.

7. *Internal and external partnership development.* Organizations that build strong internal and external alliances will increase their overall capabilities.

8. *Corporate responsibility and citizenship.* Work toward meeting safety and legal requirements beyond mere compliance. Failure to address these issues can undermine trust and adversely affect the organization's bottom line.

9. *A focus on results.* If an organization fails to focus on results, it may get bogged down in processes and neglect to focus on strategies that are critical to success.

10. *Effective leadership.* Good leaders serve as role models by reinforcing values through their words and actions. Effective leaders "walk their talk" (Blazey, 1997, pp. 61–64).

Looking Within Ourselves to Create Change

This book was written because the authors had the good fortune to have a working relationship that successfully integrated functions of human resources and marketing. As we explored the reasons for our positive outcomes to share with others, we uncovered a variety of contributing factors. An attempt has been made to highlight and promote some different ways of looking at traditional structures within organizations. We believe there is value in reviewing successful efforts from the past while continuing to create new visions for the future.

The case studies and other examples included in the previous chapters have highlighted success stories of various organizations. The details that have not been fully itemized include the months of preparation and the awkward steps that invariably occur with change. As success stories are reviewed, the following common themes begin to emerge:

- A long-term commitment to continuous evaluation and improvement
- Providing employees with the tools and information they need in order to do their best work
- Enhancing communication throughout the organization
- Recognizing the importance to employees of balancing personal and work needs

Employees want to do a good job and be associated with a respected organization. The selected case studies demonstrate that success can be achieved if organizational leaders are willing to take the bold steps required to move beyond the basic accepted standards of performance and into the company of outstanding performers.

References

Blazey, M. "Achieving Performance Excellence." *Quality Progress*, June 1997, 30(6).

James, J. "Thinking in the Future Tense." *Healthcare Forum Journal*, Jan./Feb., 1997.

Ruark, R. "Introduction." *Something of Value*. Garden City, N.Y.: Doubleday, 1955.

Townsend, P., and Gebhardt, J. "Making Change Possible." *Journal for Quality and Participation*, Mar. 1997.

Index

A

Above & Beyond Award, *107*
Absenteeism, caused by grief, 114–115
Absenteeism rates, 7, 8, 166; reducing, 19, 115
Aburdene, P., 4, 5, 10
Abuse, 74
Academic skills, 124
Academy of Management Executive, 7
Access, reduced, 74
Accident rates, 7, 8, 156
Accountability, 48, 53, 125, 149; example of, 200–201
Acquisitions, corporate, perception of, 74, 181
Acquisitions, customer, 1, 179, 189, 193
Action items, 50
Action plans, 49, *50*, 63
Action, taking, 52, 53, 55
Actions, 31, 54, 55; alignment of, 34, 37, 47; based on personal interest, 60; consistency in, 51, 52, 55–56
Ad hoc focus groups, 82
Advancement opportunities, 14, 167; as a measure, 99, 168
Advertising, 126; costs and benefits of, 191–192; effectiveness of, 180; focus on, 40, 189; limitations of, 179; and perceptions, 74–75, 97, 181–182, 192
Advertising, word-of-mouth, 8, 40, 98–99, 101, 180, 193
Advertising-war campaigns, 192
African Basuto proverb, 205
After-school programs, 114
Age diversity, 3, 110–111
Aging, of the workforce, effects of, 122
Alexander, C. P., 91
Alignment issues, dealing with, 79–80

Allerton, H. E., 171
Alliances, internal and external, 210
"America at Work" study, 170
American Hospice Association, 114
American Hospital Association (AHA), 73, 74, 75, 181, 182, 183
American Society for Training and Development, 140
Americans with Disabilities Act, 106
Amnesia, corporate, 13
Anthem Health Systems, *164*
Aon Consulting, 170
Arthur Andersen LLP, 1, 48, 77, 115
Assertiveness skills, measuring, 129
Assets: as a measure, 76; people as, 3, 77, 142
Assumption reversal, 33
Atkinson, M., 141
Attitudes, 103–104, 130–131; measuring, 142; role of, 85; shaping of, 36
Attrition. *See* Turnover
Austin, N. K., 110, 170
Authoritarian leadership style, 61
Autonomy, as a measure, 99, 168
Avis, 116
Awards, 106, *107–109*

B

Baby boomers, 4, 111
Balanced Scorecard, The (Kaplan and Norton), 10
Balancing work and personal life, 8, 123; addressing, 10, 20–21, 170–171, 211; and flexible scheduling, 165–166; implementing programs for, 114, 170
Baptist Hospital, 198–203
Basile, F., 104
Battistella, R., 160

Beckham, D., 51

Behavior, *59*, 104; disruptive, 57, *59*; nonverbal, 129; positive, 54, 55, 106, 169; as the product, 71

Behavioral coaching, 196

Behavioral expectations, 104–105, 145–148

Behavioral interview questions, 128–129, 130–131

Behavioral Trust and Change Program, 58, *59*

Bellandi, D., 191

Benchmarking, 103, 116–117, 136; source for, 209; and training, 142, 152, 153

Benefits, 1, 11, 87, 169; changes in, 160–167; competitive, 159; unique, examples of, *165, 170. See also specific types*

Benefits, health, 160–161, 164–165

Billboards, 191

"Bizarro," 14

Blalock, T., 111

Blazey, M., 211

Blood pressure/glucose, 163

Bloom, J., 195

Board member involvement, 12–13, 25, 26, 32, 35, 49

Bond, J. T., 168

Bonus checks, 68, 101, 102, 126

Boylan, B., 30, 36

Brochures, use of, 189, 191, 193

Built to Last: Successful Habits of Visionary Companies (Collins and Porras), 13, 34, 37, 47, 52, 57, 61

Burchfield, D., 160

Burnout, 171

Buyer's market, 4

C

Cadena, C., 202

Care, clinical, 3

Career survival, 19

Carmichael, B., 154

Case, J., 149

Catlette, B., 85

Cerrato, P. L., 164

Change: barriers to, 209; and chaos, 31; courage to, 19; fear of, 205, 209; and Generation X employees, 110; guidelines for, 205–206; need for, 31; perceptions of, 29, 74; and reengineering, 148–149; resistance to, *34, 35, 42*; support for, 184; and transition, 205; and use of focused dialogue, 172

Change agents, 58

Child care, 101, 113, 114, 122, 166–167

Cigna Corporation, *165*

Cinergy Services, Inc., 38

Circle of Quality Service award, 176

Clarian Health Partners, 39, 40, 43

Clarification, *52*

Clinical outcomes, 2, *3*, 18, 90

Cobb, J. C., 80, 84, 85, 92, 97, 172

Code of conduct, 65

Collaboration, departmental, 84

Collaboration leadership style, 61

Collaborative traits, developing, 55

College courses, offering, 141, 152–153

Collins, J. C., 13, 38, 47, 48, 57, 61

Commitment, 14, 92, 127, 206; to strategic plans, 51, *52*, 53

Commitment, employer, 98

Communication: enhancing, 206, 211; language in, 183; as a survey topic, 153; verbal, preference for, 186

Communication sessions, 64

Communication skills, 105–106, 124, 129, 186

Communications: external, 189–193, 191, 198; internal, 80, 81–82, 184–189, 190, 206, 211. *See also specific mediums*

Community expectations, 6

Community involvement, 86, 123–124

Community needs, meeting, 179

Community perceptions, 73–75, 86–87, 174, 194

Compassion, example of, 173

Competency: basic, 139, 141, 142, 151; core, 87–88, 135; technical, 74, 103, 125, 154–157, 182

Competition: differentiation from, 30, 78, 79; for first-rate employees, 4, 5, 98

Competitive edge, 14, 31, 72; sources of, 5, 7, 86

Competitive wages, 159

Competitiveness, 55, 196

Confidence gap, 184

Confidentiality, 164

Conflict, 25, 156

Conflict management skills, measuring, 129

Congressional Budget Office, 160

Congruity, 38

Connectedness, 52
Connors, R., 149
Constancy, 38
Constraint removal, 33
Consultants, use of, 144
Consumers. *See* Customers
Contented Cows Give Better Milk (Catlette and Hadden), 85
Continuing education, 118; on-site, offering, 140, 141, 152–153. *See also* Education programs; Learning opportunities
Continuous evaluation, 210, 211
Continuous learning, as a measure, 110
Continuous quality improvement (CQI), 85, 91, 104, 146; commitment to, 103, 210, 211; example of, 176–177; focus on, 40
Contract employment, 1
Control, 52
Coors wellness program, *164*
Coping skills, measuring, 128
Core business. *See* Mission, vision, and values
Core purpose. *See* Mission
Corporatization, effect of, 6, 74, 182
Cost containment, 1
Cost savings, 141, 156
Costs, rising, 1, 74, 192
Counseling programs, 114
Covey, S. R., 32, 139
Creativity skills, measuring, 129
Cross-selling, 87
Cross-training, 93, 111
Cultural barriers, 106
Cultural competence assessment, 117, 118
Customer acquisition, 1, 179, 189, 193
Customer Comes Second, The (Rosenbluth and Peters), 103, 135
Customer dissatisfaction, 182, 210
Customer expectations, 78, 80, 104, 183, 185
Customer loyalty, 9
Customer needs: identifying, 189; taking care of, 79, 80, 86, 173
Customer newsletters, 189, 193
Customer orientation, 40
Customer perceptions, 71; and advertising, 74–75, 97, 181–182, 192; of organizations, 2, 181–183; and value, 90
Customer preference, assumptions about, 79

Customer relations council, 86
Customer retention, 76, 179, 189, 196
Customer satisfaction, 2, 4, 90; effects on, 8–9, 21, 84; improving, model for, 199–203; investment in, 76–77; as a measure, 76; measuring, 200, 201
Customer satisfaction surveys, 78, 156, 195, 196–197
Customer service: addressing, 65, 146; in defining quality, 79; definitions for, discussion of, 37; developing excellence in, 196; measuring success of, 118; and performance appraisals, 79; standards for, defining, 78; and training, 141; and value, 90
Customer service excellence, 40, 77, 78–79
Customer service measures, 201
Customer service skills, 105–106, 125, 196
Customer service training programs, 78, 197
Customer volume, improving, 194
Customers, 13, 29, 80–81; defining, 81; employees as, 44; hired as employees, 173, 197; importance of, 2, 3, 10
Customers, internal. *See* Employees

D

Data availability, 210
"Data Watch," 191
Day care centers, on-site, 114, 166
Day care information, providing, 166–167
DeBecker, G., 131, 134
Decision making, 25, 47, 67, 209, 210; assisting operational departments with, 195–196; compassion in, 173–174; and empowerment, 148–149; example of, 203; factors affecting, 60; guidance for, 29, 30–31, 173–174; independent, 65; and information flow, 53; sharing, 13
Decision-making authority, 168
Decision-making errors, 66
Decision-making skills, measuring, 129
Delegation, 75
Demographic data, use of, 122, 189–190
Demographics, 20, 112, 113
Denial, 75
Dependent care. *See* Child care; Elder care

Depression, 163
Development. *See* Performance development; Personal development
"Dilbert," 14, 53
Direct mail, 191
Disability, 112
Disney, 145
Disney model, example of, 116–119
Distance learning programs, 152–153
Diversity action council, 117
Diversity issues, 106, 110–112, 209
Dollar capital, 5
Donors, 5, 187, 197
Drennan, D., 180
Drucker, P., 53
DYG, Inc., 48, 77

E

Economist, The, 17
Education, and diversity, 112
Education programs, 58, 106, 110, 118. *See also* Continuing education; Learning opportunities
Efficiency measures, example of, 201
eHealth, 64
E.I. du Pont de Nemours Company, 167
Einstein, K., 129
Elder care, 113, 114, 122, 166
Electronic Data Systems, 9
Eli Lilly and Company, 20–21
Ellig, B. R., 135
E-mail, use of, 188
Employee assistance plans (EAPs), 114, 115
Employee dissatisfaction, 5, 8
Employee handbook, 64, 65, 68
Employee needs, responding to, 80, 167, 168–169
Employee newsletters, 184, 185, 186
Employee of the Month, *107–108*
Employee relations councils, 82, *107–108*
Employee satisfaction, 3, 16–17, 88, 168, 193; effects of, 6, 7–9, 21, 84; factors in, 11, 99–100, 102, 123, 168; improving, 169, 199–203; increasing, 2, 115, 161; as a measure, 76; measuring, 9, 153–154; supporting, 84, 85, 86
Employee satisfaction data, use of, 9
Employee satisfaction surveys, 44, 156
Employee selection. *See* Hiring; Interviewing

Employees, 63; as customers, 44, 80–81, 115; defined, 18; importance of, 2, 3, 5, 10; priorities of, 99–100, 171; prospective, 58, 98, 101–102, 128, 130. *See also* Workforce, the
Employer-of-choice reputation, 20–21, 88, 126. *See also* Work environments, positive
Employment relationships, 11, 12
Employment trends, 103, 152
Empowerment, 148–149, 209, 211
Endorsements, use of, 142, 193
ER–7 emergency department, 194–195
Evaluations, employee. *See* Performance appraisals
Exchange meetings, 59
Executive search firms, use of, 127
Exit interviews, 117
Expense management measures, 201
Expenses, as a measure, 76
"Eye on Patients" survey, 182

F

Facilitators, 49, 144, 156, 157
Families and Work Institute study, 99
Fear, 60, 205, 209
Fellers, G., 60
Financial assets, 77
Financial bottom line, 74
Financial compensation, 1, 68, 147, 201; in recruiting, 101, 102, 126. *See also* Wages
Financial performance, 7, 15; as a by-product, 13; effects on, 6, 8–9; shifting focus from, 77. *See also* Profits
Financial security, corporate, 85–86
Firing, reasons for, 104
1st Community Bank and Trust, 92–95
Fitness centers, 115
Flexibility skills, measuring, 129
Flexible health benefits, 164–165
Flexible scheduling, 165–166; for dependent care, 167; and Generation X employees, 21; as a job quality measure, 102; offering, 126, 140, 161; options for, 113
Flexible spending accounts, 164, 166
Focus group interviews, 124
Focus groups, 82, 159
Focus on Health, 107
Focused dialogue technique, 172

Ford, K., 140
For-profit organizations, 5–6
Fortune, 135
Franklin Community School Corpora-
    tion, 124
Franklin Research and Development, 7
Fraud, 74
Fulfilling work, 122–123
Fulghum, R., 38
Future, 31, 32–33, 54, 208–209, 210

G

Gainsharing program, 177
Galinsky, E., 168
Gallup Organization surveys, 9, 16, 123,
    182, 191
Gardner, J., 182
Gebhardt, J., 205
Gender, and diversity, 112
Generation X employees, 4, 21, 98,
    110–111
Generational differences, 3, 110, 112
*Get Everyone in your Boat Rowing in the
    Same Direction: 5 Leadership Principles
    to Follow So Others Will Follow You*
    (Boylan), 36
Giller, D., 195
Goals. *See* Organizational goals; Personal
    goals; Strategic goals
Goal-setting skills, measuring, 128
Goeb, D., 92–95
Goetzel, R. Z., 163
*Great Place to Work, A: What Makes Some
    Employers So Good (And Most So Bad)*
    (Levering), 7, 14
Grief and terminal illness counseling,
    114–115
Grief at Work, 114
Grievances filed, 7, 8
Guest relations training program,
    174–178

H

Hacker, C. A., 121, 128, 132
Hadden, R., 85
Hamilton, L., 111
Hard factors, 11, 15
Harriman, B., 203
HCA Wesley, 39
"Healing Healthcare" management team,
    157

Health 2000, 143
Health benefits, 160–161, 164–165
Health care costs, rising, 160–161
Health care industry: as a business of rela-
    tionships, 115–116; view of, 1–2, 182
Health care organizations: corporatization
    of, 6, 74, 182; defined, 18; future of,
    208–209; measuring, 11, 15; new pres-
    sures facing, 3–5; selection of, 180;
    view of, 1, 88
Health Direct, 64
Health Enhancement Research Organiza-
    tion (HERO) database, 162–163
Health Forum, 48, 77
Health insurance coverage, 160–161
Health promotion, 161–164, *165*; focus
    on, 115–116, 122
Health Risk Appraisal (HRA), 162
Health risk factors, 163
Heeley, G. F., 38, 58
Henkoff, R., 104
Hequet, M., 76, 77
Herman, R. E., 159, 167
Heroic behavior, 12, 62
Heroic environment, principles of, 12
Hickman, C., 149
Himmelman, A., 58
Hiring, 93, 124, 125; bad decisions in,
    121; and developing core competen-
    cies, 87–88, 135; importance of, 3, 54,
    136–137; of replacement workers, cost
    of, 5, 8, 89; the right employees,
    71–72, 97, 103–104, 135–137. *See also*
    Interviewing
Hiring, from within, 13, 14, 62, 89, 127
Hiring process, 117; example of, 135–137
Hobart, A., 111
Hochstein, M., 48
Honesty, 55
Hospital Happenings, *107*, *108*
Housecleaning incentive, 101
Howgill, M.W.C., 39–43
Human capital, 5
"Human Resources and the Bottom Line"
    (Zigarelli), 7
Human Resources Development Hall of
    Fame, 142
Human resources functions: change in
    perspective of, 41; definitions of, 18,
    73, 97; role of, 72, 77, 78, 80, 196. *See
    also* Integration, of human resources
    and marketing functions

Human resources staff: experience of, 73; lack of understanding in, 83–84; methods used by, 82–83; view of, 83
Human touch, the, 71

I

Image. *See* Employee image; Organizational image
Immerwarh, J., 16
Impersonal care, 74
"Improving Organization Performance" standard, 90
Inaction, 55
Inc., 199
Incentives. *See specific types*
Indiana University Hospital (IU), 43
Inflation, 1
Information, free flow of, 53, 86–87
Information society, 3, 4, 5
Inforum, 191
Initiative skills, measuring, 129
Inside McMurry, 57
Insurers, and health promotion, 162
Integration, of human resources and marketing functions: benefits of, 18–19, 63, 84–89; a case study in, 40–44; defined, 2, 3; models for, 90–95; overview of steps to, 207; reactions to, 206. *See also* Human resources functions; Marketing functions
Integrity, 38, 51
Intellectual capital, 76, 196
Intelligence, expanding, 209
Internet, use of the: by day care centers, 166–167; for distance learning programs, 153; as an employment source, 98; as a recruiting tool, 126, 170, 189
Interview teams, 132–134
Interviewing: behavioral questions for, 128–129, 130–131; examples of, 136, 137; follow-up to, 134–135; preparing for, 121, 128–134, 145. *See also* Hiring
Interviewing skills, teaching, 177
Intranet, use of, 188
Intuit, 165
"It's the Manager, Stupid," 17

J

Jackson, J. H., 7
Jacobson, D., 99
James, J., 208

Jamieson, D., 112, 113, 122
Jesus, CEO (Jones), 60
Job descriptions, 104, 105, 135
Job fairs, 126–127
Job performance. *See* Performance
Job satisfaction. *See* Employee satisfaction
Job security, as a measure, 99, 102, 168
Job sharing, 113, 161, 167
Johnson Memorial Hospital, 105–106; award programs, 107–109
Joint Commission on Accreditation of Healthcare Organizations (JCAHO), 89–90, 104, 106, 151, 156
Jones, L. B., 60
Jones, P., 25–26
Journey into the Heroic Environment, A (Lebow), 12
Just, J., 148

K

Kahaner, L., 25–26
Kaiser, L., 31, 32, 33, 34, 52, 54, 208
Kaplan, R., 10
Kelley, S., 161
Kennedy, C., 102
Key Contributor Award, 107, 108
Kiser, K., 142
Knowledge Soft, 144
Kotter, J. P., 30, 31, 35, 184
Kreuter, M., 143
Kupperschmidt, B. R., 98, 111

L

Laabs, J., 167, 170
Lands' End, 167
Lange, C., 20–21
Language gap, 83, 183
Layoffs, 1
Leader, defined, 57
Leaders: qualities needed in, 35, 38, 60–61; responsibilities of, 58; strategic, 51; visionary, 47, 57
Leadership: effective, 60–61, 211; restructuring, 90–91
Leadership development, investing in, 58
"Leadership for a Healthy 21st Century" study, 48, 77
Leadership issues, 58
Leadership Moment, The (Useem), 13
Leadership retreats, 49
Leadership skills, measuring, 128

Leadership styles, 61
Learning opportunities, 99, 140; as a measure, 99, 102, 110, 123, 168. *See also* Continuing education; Education programs
Leaving. *See* Turnover
Lebow, R. A., 12, 15
Lee, C., 98
Lee Hecht Harrison, 102
Leonard, B., 102
Leverence, J., 150
Levering, R. A., 7, 10–11, 12, 14, 15
Liabilities, as a measure, 76
Licensing organizations, requirements of, 140
Lifestyle, and diversity, 112
Losey, D., 98, 100
Losey, M., 99
Loveday, B., 40–41, 43–44
Loyalty, 14, *53*, 85, 111, 170; and job quality measures, 99–100
Lyons, N. J., 199–203

M

Mackay, H. B., 129
MacStravic, S., 198
Magazines, use of, 189, 191, 193
Malcolm Baldrige Quality award, 209–210
Management: credibility in, 35; educational background of, 15; responsibilities of, defined, 3; success in, 60–61
Management Review, 76
Manager, defined, 57
Manager training, 167
Marketing: definition of, 72, 179; under-valuing, 44
Marketing budgets, 19
Marketing fair, 189
Marketing functions: defined, 17–18, 73, 82; role of, 78, 79–80, 196. *See also* Integration, of human resources and marketing functions
Marketing mediums. *See specific types*
Marketing staff: focus of, 44; lack of understanding in, 83–84; methods of, 82–83; view of, 83
Massage therapy, *165*
Master's programs, limitations of, 15
Matejka, K., 13, 51, 53, 57, 58
Maternity leave, 113

Mathis, R. L., 7
Mayo, E., 85
McDonald, T., 140, 142
McGill, M., 91
MCI, 5
McMurry, C. M., 64–65, 66–67
McMurry, P., 56–57, 63, 64, 65, 66, 68, 136–137
McMurry Publishing, Inc., 56, 63–68, 136–137
McVeigh, P., 7
Meaningful work, 11, 123; as a measure, 99, 168
Measurement model, 77
Medical expense averages, 163
Medical savings accounts, 160–161
MEDSTAT Group, 162
Memorial Hospital, *165*
Mentors, use of, 146–148, 186
Mercer, W. M., 113, 114
Mergers, perception of, 74, 181
Merit pay system, 41
Metaphors, creating new, 33
Methodist Hospital of Indiana, Inc., 39–43
Micco, L., 9, 123
Micromanagement leadership style, 61
Mission, 34, 81; defined, 24; living the, example of, 63–68; placing priority on, 104–105; supporting, 37, 78, 98; tradi-tional, 73
Mission statements, 28, 66, 181, 207–208; components of, 24–25; creating, 25–26, *27*
Mission, vision, and values, 6, 13, 38, 58; adherence to, 34; changes in, 13; con-sistency in, 13; defined, 2; ensuring compatibility with, 47; forgetting, 6, 13; fulfilling, difficulty in, 52; role of, 39; success in defining, 48
Mission, vision, and values statements, 55, 135; defining key words in, 47; use of, 23–24; uselessness of, 39
Monday morning meetings, 64–65
Monitoring behavior, 59
Morale, enhancing, 127
Morgan, R. B., 127, 128, 134, 135
Motivation, 13, 99, 125, 168; analyzing, 59, 85; assessing, 103; enhancing, 127, 196; role of vision in, 30, 31; sustaining, 114
Motivational posters, use of, 187
Motivations, shifting, 122
Motorola, 116

"Mouseker Award," 116
Mycek, S., 2, 48, 116, 135
Mythology, corporate, 52–53, 62
Myths, recognizing, 209

N

Naisbitt, J., 4, 5, 10
National Research Corporation, 180
National Study of the Changing Workforce (1997), 160, 168
New product development, as a measure, 76
New services development, 195–196
Newcomer programs, 193
Newspaper advertisements, 126, 191
Nominal group process, use of, 50
Nonprofit organizations, 5–6
Northern Telecom, 9
Nurses, and quality definitions, 181
Nursing orientation session, 172–173

O

Objectives, 23, 36, 48, 49, 51
Occupational Safety and Health Administration (OSHA), 139, 151
Officer call program, 93
O'Mara, J., 112, 113, 122
"100 Best Companies to Work for in America" list, 7, 135
One-to-one marketing, 197
On-the-job socialization, 62, 100, 146
Open-book management (OBM) program, 67–68
Operational departments: assisting, 2, 78, 88, 193–196; input from, lack of, 62
Opinion Research Corporation International, 191
ORC Health Care, 191
Organizational chart, traditional, 73
Organizational culture, 42, 169; articulating, 25; challenging, risks in, 58; changing, examples of, 174–178, 198–203; creating, and values, 36; definition of, 135; describing, with stories, 52–53; effect of group communication on, 82; fitting into, 117; as an obstacle, 34, 35; perception of, 159; preferred, creating, 58
Organizational development (OD) concept, 91
Organizational goals, 25; achieving, 23, 47, 84, 118; action items and, 50;
aligning training with, 145; alignment with, 72; attainable, choosing, 28–29; commitment to, 52, 53; communicating, 81; driving, 49; time-specific, 31; and training, 141; understanding, 23, 189. See also Strategic goals
Organizational image, 18, 86, 101, 193; and alignment, 79–80; factors involved in, 2, 3; lasting impressions of, 134; perception versus reality of, 190; perceptions of, 180–183, 190, 192
Organizational needs, focus on, 80
Organizational performance, 2, 3–4, 7, 14, 44, 91; and standards, 49; standards for improving, 89–90
Organizational performance measures, 76, 77
Organizational structures, as an obstacle, 34, 35
Organizing skills, measuring, 129
Orientation, 64, 145–148, 177, 185–186; lack of structured approach to, 140; for students, 100
Orientation plan, use of, 137
Outcomes, clinical, 2, 3, 18, 90
Oz Principle, The (Connors, Smith, and Hickman), 149

P

Parry, S., 142
Passive leaders, 58
Paternity leave, 113
Patients. *See* Customers
Peer coaches, 156, 157
Penson, P. G., 153
People-Centered Teams: Healing the Workplace program, 154–157
Perception versus reality, 181–182
Performance, 2, 3, 19; effects on, 6, 9, 14, 16–17; focus on, 44; improving, 2; loss of, 8; poor, reason for, 42; raising, 16; reevaluating ideas on, 3; and standards, 79
Performance appraisal process: example of, 66–67
Performance appraisal systems, 79, 125, 176
Performance appraisals, 41, 104, 105, 148, 201; and cultural competence, 117; example of, in management, 201; focus of, 151; instilling values through, 177

Performance development, 140, 141–142; approaches to, 139, *152*; assessing need for, 151–152; example of, in management, 200; goals of, 147, 150–151. *See also* Training

Performance development programs, 117, 119, 154–157. *See also* Training programs

Performance, financial. *See* Financial performance

Performance indicators, 59

Performance issues, caused by grief, 114–115

Performance measurements, linking, to strategy, 18

Performance, organizational. *See* Organizational performance

Personal development, 126, 151, 153

Personal goals, 72, 148, 151

Personal interest, 60

Personal issues, addressing, 113

Personality traits, 103–104

Perspectives, changing, 33

Peters, D. M., 97, 135, 136

Peters, T., 177–178

Physical assets, 77

Physicians, 49; as employees, 2, 18, 187–188

Picker Institute, 182

Pinsker, R. J., 127

Piraro, D., 14

Policies, 11, 17, 36, 173–174; creating, defined, 49; defining terms in, 150

Politics, internal, 17, 60

Porras, J. I., 13, 38, 47, 48, 57, 61

Power struggles, 55

Praxis, defined, 38

Preceptors, use of, 146–148, 150, 186

President's Quality Council, 176

Press, Ganey Associates, Inc., 196

Prevention, of illness. *See* Health promotion

Pride, 12

Procedures, 36, 173–174; defined, 49

Process implementation, evaluating, 82

Productivity. *See* Performance

Profit margin, as a measure, 76

Profit maximization, 15

Profit sharing, 67, 68

Profits, 5, 182; increase in, 6, 67; maximizing, 15–16, 18, 19. *See also* Financial performance

Programs, defined, 49

Promises, 59

Promoting employees. *See* Hiring, from within

Promotional campaigns, 193

Provider, health care. *See* Health care organizations

Provider-of-choice reputation, gaining, 88

Psychologist, corporate, use of, 136

Public. *See* Community entries

Punishments, 57, 59, 62

"Putting the Work Ethic to Work" (Yankelovich and Immerwahr), 16

Q

Quality decline, customer belief in, 182

Quality of care, 74, 182, 183–184; defining, 79, 181, 183; focus on, 40; as a measure, 76

Quality outcomes, 18

R

Race, and diversity, 112

Ratio, as a measure, 76

"Reality √" (American Hospital Association), 73–74, 75, 181–182, 183, 192

"Reality √ II" (American Hospital Association), 74–75, 181–182

Recognition, 14, 122, 123, 153, 168; example of, 201–202; need for, 11, 126, 175; suggestions for, 175–176; uses of, *53*, 58, 206. *See also* Rewards

Recognition awards, 106, *107–109*

Recruiting, 4, 19, 87; consistent messages in, 190; difficulties in, 1, 8, 88, 89, 98; enhancing, 124, 154, 170; focus on, 40; improving, 154; of replacement workers, cost of, 8; sources used for, 126–128; of students, benefits of, 100–101; and training, 140, 141; use of demographic data in, 122; using incentives in, 101–102, 126, 159; and word-of-mouth advertising, 98–99

Reengineering, focus on, 148–149

References, checking, 134

Regrouping, 59

Regulatory agency requirements, 139, 140, 142, 151

"Reinventing Methodist" program, 42

Re-inventing the Corporation (Naisbitt and Aburdene), 4

Relationships, importance of, 115–116, 154, 196, 197–198

Reliability, 38
Religious barriers, 106
Relocation, 122
Resources, 2, 5, 58
Respect, for abilities, 53
Respectful treatment, 11
Responsibility, 53, 125
Responsibility, corporate, 210
Restructuring, 1, 40, 90–91
Results, focus on, 210
Résumés, 132, 134
Retention, 3, 9, 87, 98–99; difficulty of, 1, 88, 98; improving, 154, 170; incentives for, 161; investment in, 76–77; and job quality measures, 99–100; as a measure, 76; of the right employees, 71–72; and training, 140, 141. *See also* Turnover
Retention, customer. *See* Customer retention
Retention rate, improved, 118
Return on investment, as a measure, 76
Revenue, as a measure, 76
Reward systems, 34, 35, 55, 122, 153
Rewarding behaviors, 54–55, 59, 106, 169
Rewards, 84; example of, 201–202; for preceptors, 147; use of, 53, 176. *See also* Recognition
Rewards, monetary. *See* Financial compensation
Reynolds Electrical & Engineering Company, Inc., *164*
Riley Hospital for Children, 43
Risk managers, 149
Risk taking, 19, 149, 202
Risky Business Award, *109*
Ritz-Carlton Hotel, 116
Robinson, D. G., 151
Robinson, J. C., 151
Role models, 156, 175; importance of, 97, 125, 211
Rosenbluth, H. F., 97, 103–104, 135, 136
Rosenbluth Travel, 135–136
Ruark, R., 205
Rules, breaking, example of, 202
Russell, L., 76

S

Sabbaticals, 122
St. Charles Medical Center, 154–157

Salary. *See* Wages
Sales training, 93
Samuel, C. J., 80, 84, 85, 92, 97, 172
Satisfaction. *See* Customer satisfaction; Employee satisfaction
Say It and Live It: 50 Corporate Mission Statements That Hit the Mark (Jones and Kahaner), 25–26
Scheduling, flexible. *See* Flexible scheduling
School-to-work programs, 101, 124
Scoring grid, use of, 133
Screen savers, use of, 188
Sears Roebuck, 9
Securities and Exchange Commission, 76
Sedentary lifestyle, 163
Self-fulfilling prophecy, 54
Senge, P. M. (and others), 35
Service. *See* Customer service
Service economy, 3, 4
Seven C's of strategic commitment, 52
Seven Habits of Highly Effective People, The (Covey), 139
Sexton, M. W., 80, 84, 85, 92, 97, 172
Shadowing, use of, 101, 126, 176
SHARE Program, *107, 109*
Shareholders. *See* Stockholders
Sharkproof (Mackay), 129
Shellenbarger, S., 5, 8–9, 10
Sick days, 19, 161
Sign-on bonuses, 101, 102, 126
Sinai Hospital, 194–195
Skills assessment counseling, 114
Smart Health, 64
Smith, J. E., 127, 128, 134, 135
Smith, T., 149
Smoldt, R. K., 180
Social change, 4
Social skills, 125
Society for Human Resource Management, 9, 99
Soft factors, 11, 15
Soft skills, 103, 105, 118, 142
Something of Value (Ruark), 205
Speaking, with consistency, 51, 52, 54
Stakeholders, 5–6, 12–13
Stamps, D., 144, 151
Standard and Poor's 500, 7
Status quo, 35, 184
Stay Well Company, The, 162
Still, D. J., 131, 132
Stockholders, 5–6, 12–13, 15, 16, 29

Strategic commitment process, 52
Strategic goals, 139, 141, 145, 206–207; defining, 48, 49. *See also* Organizational goals
Strategic planning process, 49–51
Strategies, 25, 59; developing, 49, 50–51, 62–63
Strategy, 18, 23, 47, 48, 85; and addressing diversity, 117; commitment to, *51, 52, 53*
Strategy development session, questions for, *50*
Stress, 19, 114, 161, 163, 166; increased, 171; and lack of control, 21
Stress management, 114, 115, *164, 165*
Student loan payoff, 101
Studer, Q., 199–203
Success, 58, *59,* 72, 76; long-term, 139; measuring, 68, 77, 118
Success measures, 118
Summer camp programs, 114
Surveying, 20, 21, 152, 153–154, 159
Swanberg, J., 168
Swartz, D., 202

T

T.E.A.M. Committee, *107, 109*
Team interviews, structuring, 132–134
Team-building skills, measuring, 129
Teamwork, 13, 21, 55
Teamwork survey, 68
Technical competency, 74, 103, 125, 154–157, 182
Technical courses, on-site, 141
Technology, new, pressures from, 3
Television advertisements, 191
Terminology, defining, 150, 207–208
Testimonials, use of, 127, 142
Texas Instruments, 167
Thurow, L. C., 9–10, 13–14, 15–16
Time off, 113, 122, 147
Tobacco use, 163
Todd, A., 144
Towner-Larsen, B., 148
Townsend, P., 205
Traditionalists, 111
Trainers, internal versus external, 144–145
Training, 3, 93, 151, 153, 167; aligning, 145; approaches to, 139, *152;* commitment to, 140–141; difficulty in, 1; elim-
inating, 141; focus of, 144; focus on, 40; importance of, 19, 71–72; as a measure, 76; measurement standards for, 79; of replacement workers, cost of, 5, 8. *See also* Performance development
Training House, Inc., 142
Training needs, defining, 143
Training programs, 174–178; in customer service, 78, 197; implementing, 58; justifying, 141–142; measuring success of, 119; for preceptors, 147; to reinforce communications, 186–187; visionary, 62. *See also* Performance development programs
Transition, dealing with, 205, 208
Trust, 6, 12, 175, 210; in change, 206; developing, 38, 58, *59,* 92, 175; embracing, 55; lack of, 55–56, 61, 75, 84, 202; regaining, 76, 184; undermining, 61
Tuition reimbursement, 126, 140
Turf protection, 84, 92
Turnover, 1, 9, 10; cost of, 8, 161; and diversity issues, 110; measures of, example of, 201; rate of, 7, 8, 102, 118, 119; reasons for, 10, 99–100, 102, 127, 167; reduced, 6, 68; reducing, 19, 105. *See also* Retention

U

UCH Academy, 117
Unemployment rates, 4
University of Chicago Hospitals system, 116–119
University of Texas MD Anderson Cancer Center, The, 43
Untapped option model, 2, 3
Untapped option, the. *See* Integration, of human resources and marketing functions
U.S. News and World Report, 116
Useem, M., 13

V

Vacation time, 161
Vallerga, L., 154
Value, corporate, 90, 128, 196; measurements of, 76, 77
Values, 34, 55, 177; conflicting, 48; conveying, 102, 104, 106; defined, 24; defining, 36–37, 38, 64–65;

implementing, example of, 56–57; placing priority on, 104–105; practicing, 54, 63–68; reinforcement of, 211
Values, personal, 98
Values statements, 66, 135; creating, 36–37; follow-through of, 12–13, 17
Vim & Vigor, 64, 65
Violence, concerns about, 134
Virtual businesses, setting up, 67–68
Vision, 47; becoming reality, 207; changes in, example of, 39–43; characteristics of, 28–31; commitment to, 98; defined, 24, 26, 28; letting go of, 34; managing, 55; sabotaging, 185; communicating too little about, 184–185; and values supporting, 37
Vision statements: clearly defined, benefits of, 207–208; creating, 28, 32–35
Visionary companies, 34, 47–48, 52, 62, 178; myth about, 37–38
Visionary leaders, 47, 57
Volunteers, as employees, 2, 18, 82, 187, 197
Vroom, V., 7–8, 14

W

Wage budgets, 1
Wage increases, less focus on, 122
Wages, 11, 14, 15, 16, 41, 159. See also Financial compensation
Wake Street Journal, The, 177
WakeMed, 174–178
Wall Street Journal, The, 8
Wallam, S., 76
Warm body syndrome, 103
Warns, M., 195
Waste, 74
Web sites. See Internet, use of the

Weight issues, 163
Welcoming process, 146
Wellness programs. See Health Promotion
Whitley, E. M., 38, 58
William M. Mercer Inc., 163
Wittman, N., 148
Wong, B. D., 1, 115–116, 135
Woodward, N. H., 165
Word-of-mouth advertising. See Advertising, word-of-mouth
Work-based education, 141
Work environments, assessing, 11, 15
Work environments, positive, 5, 12; byproduct of, 6, 7, 13; as a competitive edge, 14; defining, 10–11; factors involved in, 168, 171; in-depth study on, 9; and measurement tools for, 15; rarity of, reasons for, 14–15, 17. See also Employer-of-choice reputation
Work ethic, belief about, 9–10
Work hours, increase in, 171
Workforce, the, 102, 113, 122; trends in, 98. See also Employees
Working from home, 113
Working Mother, 167
Working Together (Simmons and Mares), 16
Working Woman, 170

Y

Yankelovich, D., 16
Yellow pages, 191
"You Are the Difference" (YATD) training program, 174–178

Z

Zigarelli, M., 7